FITNESS
FOR
EVERYONE

The Prevention Total Health System®

FITNESS
FOR
EVERYONE

by the Editors of
Prevention® Magazine

 Rodale Press, Emmaus, Pennsylvania

Printed in the United States of America
on recycled paper containing a high percentage
of de-inked fiber.

**Library of Congress Cataloging
in Publication Data**
Main entry under title:

Fitness for everyone.

(The Prevention total health system)
Includes index.
1. Exercise. 2. Physical fitness. 3. Health.
I. Prevention (Emmaus, Pa.) II. Series.
RA781.F56   1984   613′.7   83-27037
ISBN 0-87857-467-0 hardcover
  4 6 8 10 9 7 5 3   hardcover

NOTICE

This book is intended as a reference volume
only, not as a medical manual or guide to self-
treatment. If you suspect that you have a medical
problem, we urge you to seek competent medical
help. Keep in mind that exercise and nutritional
needs vary from person to person, depending on age,
sex and health status. The information here is
intended to help you make informed decisions about
your health, not as a substitute for any treatment
that may have been prescribed by your doctor.

The Prevention Total Health System®
Series Editors: William Gottlieb, Mark Bricklin
Fitness for Everyone Editor: Debora Tkac
Writers: William Gottlieb (Chapter 1),
    Lewis Vaughn (Chapter 2),
    Mark Bricklin (Chapter 4),
    Nicholas S. Yost (Chapters 6, 9),
    Sharon Faelten (Chapter 7),
    Stefan Bechtel (Chapters 8, 11),
    Cathy Perlmutter (Chapter 10).
    Also, Freda Christie, Susan DeMark,
        Ardy Friedburg, Marcia Holman, Carol Keough,
        Stephen Williams
Research Chief: Carol Baldwin
Assistant Research Chief, Prevention Health Books:
    Christy Kohler
Researchers: Holly Clemson, Susan Nastasee, Carol
    Pribulka, Joann Williams, Martha Capwell, David
    Palmer, Carole Rapp, Janice Saad, Nancy
    Smerkanich, Pam Uhl, Susan Zarrow
Fitness Consultants: Budd Coates, George Hummel
Series Art Director: Jerry O'Brien
Art Production Manager: Jane C. Knutila
Designers: Lynn Foulk, Alison Lee
Illustrators: Susan M. Blubaugh, Joe Lertola, Anita
    Lovitt, Donna Ruff
Project Assistants: Tom Chinnici, John Pepper
Director of Photography: T. L. Gettings
Photo Editor: Margaret Skrovanek
Photographic Stylists: Renee R. Grimes, Scott Schmidt,
    J. C. Vera
Photo Librarian: Shirley S. Smith
Staff Photographers: Carl Doney, T. L. Gettings,
    Ed Landrock, Mitchell T. Mandel, Margaret
    Skrovanek, Christie C. Tito
Copy Editor: Jane Sherman
Production Manager: Jacob V. Lichty
Production Coordinator: Barbara A. Herman
Composite Typesetter: Brenda J. Kline
Production Assistant: Eileen Bauder
Office Personnel: Diana M. Gottshall, Susan Lagler,
    Carol Petrakovich, Cindy Harig, Marge Kresley

Rodale Books, Inc.
Senior Managing Editor: William H. Hylton
Copy Manager: Ann Snyder
Art Director: Karen A. Schell
Publisher: Richard M. Huttner
Director of Marketing: Pat Corpora
Business Manager: Ellen J. Greene
Continuity Marketing Manager: John Taylor

Rodale Press, Inc.
Chairman of the Board: Robert Rodale
President: Robert Teufel
Executive Vice President: Marshall Ackerman
Group Vice Presidents: Sanford Beldon
                                    Mark Bricklin
Senior Vice President: John Haberern
Vice Presidents: John Griffin
                        Richard M. Huttner
                        James C. McCullagh
                        David Widenmyer
Secretary: Anna Rodale

Contents

Make Exercise a Part of Life

Most of us know that excessive processing of foods can create nutritional deficiencies in those who aren't careful about their diets.

Fewer of us realize that equally harmful deficiencies can be created by another kind of human processing—the processing of physical work. Just as modern food processing can remove nearly all the fiber and trace minerals from the grain we eat, mechanization and automation have removed a key ingredient from work—physical exertion. The result is that many of us do not get the exercise our bodies need to be fit and healthy.

Somehow, though, there is no going back. Automation is here to stay. And so is the pursuit of fitness through consciously designed regimens of exercise. Far from being a craze, as some would have us believe, daily attention to physical exercise is the price we must pay in this computer age if we don't want our bodies to turn into software along with everything else. What we get for our effort is a new sense of vitality and a feeling of tranquility, too.

Fitness for Everyone shows us how to counterbalance the dangerous deficiencies of a no-sweat world with a personal exercise plan. You'll get many good ideas for beginning a program, improving the one you're on and preventing the injuries that come most often from doing too much too fast. You'll learn, in short, how to get going . . . but take it easy!

Executive Editor, **Prevention**® Magazine

1

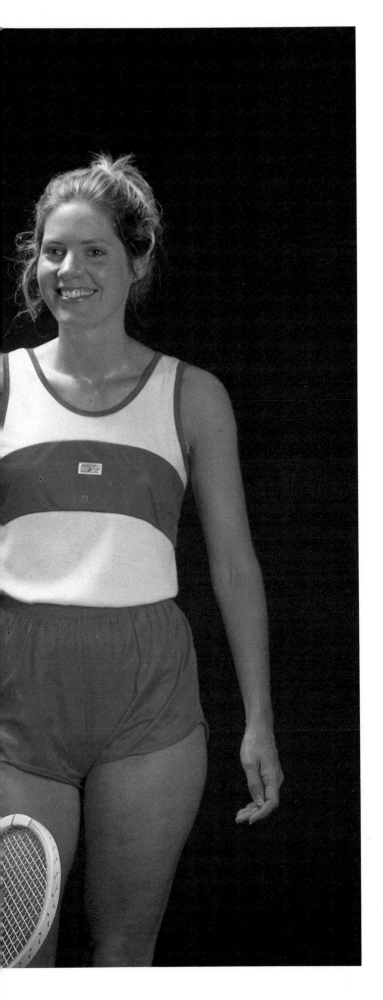

Fitness Is Health

There's a whole string of ailments that can be avoided simply by keeping the body fit.

Fitness brings the glow of good health—bright skin, lean body and energy to spare. A fit person *looks* like a healthy person. But fitness improves the way you look inside, too.

Fatty patches cling to the walls of your arteries, choking off blood to the heart. They begin to dissolve.

The arteries themselves are tightened by a clamp of tension. They loosen and relax.

Excess sugar roils through your bloodstream, a slow, sweet poison that can shorten life by 25 percent. It is sucked harmlessly into the cells.

Your skin becomes firmer, your immune system stronger, your outlook more positive . . .

You just took a miracle drug—you just took a walk around the block.

Wait a minute—a *walk* can do all that? Reverse heart disease, trim high blood pressure, help treat diabetes? We're pulling your leg, right? No, only asking you to get it moving (along with the other one, of course). Because a brisk walk—or any other kind of heart-pumping exercise you do a few times a week for at least 30 minutes a shot—can totally remodel your health. In fact, some experts say exercise is *better* than any drug.

"There is no drug in current or prospective use that holds as much promise for sustained health as a lifetime program of physical exercise," says Walter M. Bortz II, M.D., in the *Journal of the American Medical Association*.

Why is exercise so powerful? Because it's *natural*. Our bodies were made to move, and when they don't, a kind of internal rust seeps into every system and cell. Things start to clog and break down and decay. But exercise is the ultimate tune-up. It lubricates the entire body with oxygen, the oil of life. It adjusts every part of the body so that it operates at peak efficiency. And, like a master mechanic, it pays special attention to the organ that powers the entire operation—the heart.

That mechanic seems to be off duty. Heart disease kills more Americans than any other health problem—over 750,000 people every year. And the killer doesn't have just one "modus operandi." Sometimes he blocks the arteries that lead to the heart with fatty material called plaque. The flow of blood and oxygen is cut off and the muscle dies. Sometimes he forms a clot—a thrombus—that plugs up the artery like a cork in a bottle. And sometimes he panics the heart muscle into a self-destructive spasm called an arrhythmia.

But this killer is really the leader of a gang—a group of unsavory characters doctors call risk factors. They soften up a victim before the heart attack finishes him off. You might even have some of them hanging out around your body. High levels of the blood fats—cholesterol and triglycerides. High blood pressure. An impatient, overbearing, Type A personality.

Well, if risk factors are health criminals, then exercise is Wyatt Earp, the FBI and Superman all rolled into one. Numerous scientific studies have found that people who exercise reduce or get rid of their risk factors. Let's look at some of those findings, starting with the effect of exercise on blood fats.

THE TWO FACES OF CHOLESTEROL

A team of researchers checked the blood fat levels of over 7,000 men. They found that those who exercised the most (including hard physical labor outside of work) had the highest levels of cholesterol. But didn't we just finish saying that high cholesterol is a menace? Well, scientists now realize that cholesterol is a Jekyll and Hyde substance. One part of it is very good: It carries fat *away* from the arteries, and it's called high-density lipoprotein (HDL) cholesterol. The other part is very bad: It carries fat *to* the arteries, and it's called low-density lipoprotein (LDL) cholesterol. In this study, the men who got lots of exercise had average HDL cholesterol levels about 12 percent higher than those of the men who got little or no exercise. The active men also had lower LDL levels, *and* their average levels of triglycerides were 19 percent lower.

That finding would come as no surprise to Josef Patsch, M.D., a professor at Baylor College of Medicine in Houston. He's the scientist who discovered that HDL carts fat out of the blood, and he has described the blood of someone with low levels of HDL who has eaten a fatty meal as "very milky, cloudy and ugly."

Dr. Patsch tells the story of a man in a heart disease study who had very low levels of HDL and milky, fatty blood at the start of the experiment. The man became a runner, however, and when his blood

Sitting around trying to take life easy is no way to treat yourself after a heart attack. Researchers at the University of Toronto found this out after following the progress of 610 postcoronary patients over a 3-year period. They found that those who followed a regular exercise program ran only a 4.4 percent chance of having a second heart attack, compared with the 22 percent chance their less diligent counterparts faced.

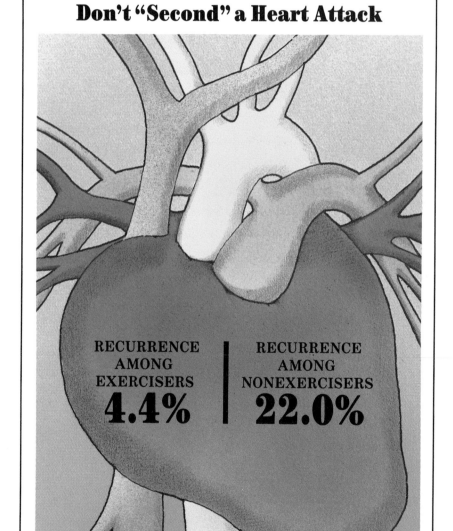

Don't "Second" a Heart Attack

RECURRENCE AMONG EXERCISERS
4.4%

RECURRENCE AMONG NONEXERCISERS
22.0%

was tested 1½ years later it was clearer. When he upped his mileage a year after that, his blood stayed perfectly clear after a fatty meal. But when a running injury forced the man to stop his exercise program for *only four weeks,* his blood turned cloudy again. Fortunately, the story has a happy—and healthy—ending. The man returned to his running program, and in six weeks his HDL was high and his blood was clear.

The moral of Dr. Patsch's story? There are two. First, he's convinced that exercise protects against heart disease by sweeping fat from food out of the blood. Second, he believes that "exercise should not be used as a medication taken only when you feel you need it. Exercise should be a lifelong habit."

SHOOTING DOWN HIGH BLOOD PRESSURE

Exercise *has* been a lifelong habit for thousands of Harvard alumni. They're part of a massive study of almost 15,000 Harvard grads from the class of 1920 through the class of 1954 whose health and exercise habits have been charted since they left college. The exercisers in the study are also the people who *don't* have a habit of getting high blood pressure (hypertension)—the tightened arteries that are major risk factors for heart disease.

"Alumni who did not engage in [vigorous exercise] were at a 35 percent greater risk of hypertension than those who did," wrote the study's scientists, who are from the Stanford University School of Medicine and the Harvard University School of Public Health.

Another scientist who has studied the link between exercise and high blood pressure is Robert Cade, M.D., a professor at the University of Florida. But Dr. Cade doesn't think exercise can just prevent high blood pressure—he thinks it can cure it.

He came to that conclusion after studying 370 people who had hypertension, measuring their blood pressure before and after fast-paced, 20-minute rides on a stationary bike.

"About 96 percent of the hypertension patients showed a significant drop in blood pressure after three months of exercising," says Dr. Cade.

Exercise, he believes, "can be an effective form of treatment for persons who suffer from hypertension, and it's also good preventive therapy for people who never want to have high blood pressure."

But what about those people who just have *pressure*? We're talking about the personalities scientists label "Type A." They think the first 2 seconds of a red light is still the caution signal, and that they have to press the elevator button three times after it's already lit. They'd sooner cut off their hand than admit they're wrong, and they're convinced that the person in an argument who shouts the loudest and bullies the most is the person who's right. They hate to lose—and they hate to see you win. In short, they're often impatient, aggressive and obnoxiously competitive.

And in a big hurry to have a heart attack.

Nobody really knows why Type A behavior causes heart disease. Maybe it's the stress hormones pumped out when a person is constantly on edge. Maybe anger clenches the arteries. But whatever is behind the problem, some scientists think they know the solution. Exercise.

A team of doctors from the Duke University Medical Center in Durham, North Carolina, studied 21 Type A personalities. At the beginning of the experiment, the study participants took a psychological test called JAS that rated the severity of their Type A characteristics. Then they joined an exercise program for ten weeks, working out three times a week for about 45 minutes a session. At the end of the ten weeks, their behavior was rated again. The group dropped from an average JAS score of 9.7 to 6.2—a major drop in impatience and aggressiveness. (That wasn't the only heart benefit. They also lowered their blood pressure, their triglycerides and their weight, and increased their HDL cholesterol.) This study, said the researchers, showed that Type A behavior "may be modified by participation in a regular exercise program."

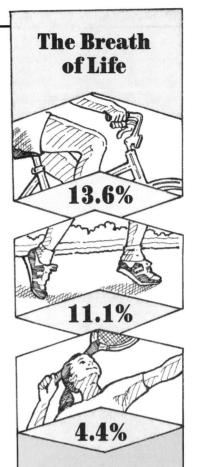

The Breath of Life

13.6%

11.1%

4.4%

One benefit of vigorous exercise is that it increases aerobic power. But not all exercises are created equal. Researchers at the University of California set out to measure the effects of 3 of the most popular exercises on maximum aerobic power and came up with these interesting percentages. After exercising 30 minutes a day 3 times a week for 20 weeks, cyclists increased their aerobic capacity the most, followed by joggers and tennis buffs.

REDUCE THE RISK OF HEART ATTACK

Okay, so exercise dissolves blood fats, grounds high blood pressure and turns a Type A into a kitten. But where's the evidence that shows it can keep you out of the Coronary Care Unit? Does any study show that an exerciser doesn't have to wonder if the guy sitting next to him on the bus knows CPR?

For the answer to that question, let's look at 572 men who did have heart attacks. They were part of a study of nearly 17,000 Harvard alumni (conducted by the same doctors who investigated the Harvard men who had high blood pressure).

The doctors divided those men into two groups—those who burned 2,000 or more calories a week in exercise, and those who burned less than 2,000.

Those who burned less got burned.

"Alumni on the low side of this index (less than 2,000 calories a week) . . . were at 64 percent increased risk of heart attack over their more energetic classmates," the researchers wrote.

What's more, they pointed out that if *all* the alumni had been in the over-2,000 category, "there would have been 86 fewer nonfatal heart attacks [and] 80 fewer fatal heart attacks, or 166 fewer than the total of 572."

The doctors were also eager to note that being a jock during college didn't protect against heart attacks in middle age—"that only a physically active adulthood is associated with lower heart attack rates." And they also said that only strenuous activities, such as jogging or swimming as opposed to bowling or golf, prevent a heart attack.

The doctors finished their report by saying that their findings "strongly support a protective role for vigorous exercise in the reduction of heart attack risk."

The verdict is in: If you don't exercise, you commit a felony against your heart. But how much exercise do you need to avoid a cardiac arrest? To find out, a team of researchers compared the risk factors of marathon runners, joggers and nonexercisers. The inactive group had higher levels of triglycerides and lower HDL cholesterol. That wasn't much of a surprise. But the next finding was that marathon runners "did not appear to be at lower risk for . . . coronary heart disease than the joggers.

"The level of physical activity necessary to reduce coronary heart disease risk probably lies between that of the joggers and the inactive men," said the researchers. "We believe that such a level of physical activity can be effectively attained without undue expenditure of time or money. Therefore, reduction of coronary heart disease risk is perhaps more within the reach of most

Exercise Doesn't Monkey Around

For several years the theory that exercise protects us from heart disease has been based on evidence that regular exercisers suffer fewer heart attacks than sedentary people. Unfortunately this evidence is what doctors call circumstantial, since differences in heredity or diet could also account for the data.

For direct proof, scientists would have to exert strict control over diet and exercise, and that's virtually impossible to do with people for any significant length of time.

Researchers at Boston University Medical Center finally got around this problem by studying monkeys. Malaysian monkeys were divided into three groups. The first group ate ordinary feed and got no exercise. The second group ate regular feed for 1 year, then switched to high-cholesterol feed for 2 years. They also got no exercise. Group 3 ate the regular diet for 18 months, then switched to a high-cholesterol diet for 2 years. They ran on treadmills in amounts equivalent to an hour of jogging 3 times a week.

Studies of the animals showed that the exercisers developed far less atherosclerosis than the sedentary monkeys, which developed considerably clogged arteries—direct physical proof that regular long-term moderate exercise can probably reduce atherosclerotic heart disease.

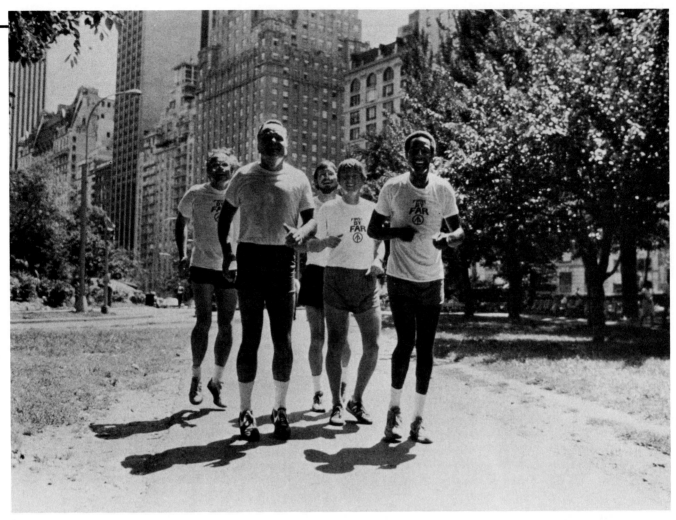

individuals than has been previously thought."

And that includes you.

THE WEIGHT LOSS FACTOR

Knowing that exercise protects against heart disease should take a load off your mind. But exercise can take a load off your body, too—the overload called fat.

Some people think exercise does just the opposite, that all that sweating and huffing and hauling yourself around turns the appetite control to *gorge*. Well, that idea is about as sensible as most diets. In one study, for example, researchers took a close look at the effect of moderate exercise on the eating habits of three obese women who had checked into a hospital for what they were told were "metabolic studies."

For the first five days, the women did no exercise at all while their daily food consumption was secretly monitored. Then, for the

next two months, they worked out each day on a treadmill. Their exercise programs were individually tailored, becoming steadily more difficult as they got into shape, so that they would burn the same amount of energy each day for the entire study period. Throughout all this, the scientists provided them with unlimited amounts of tasty but simple food—while they secretly made note of every crumb that disappeared from their plates.

Results? Despite their daily workouts, the women continued to eat about the same amount of food as they had when they were exercising nothing but their minds. And since their daily bouts with the treadmill burned more energy, they all started losing weight.

"Obese women doing long-term moderate exercise do not compensate by an increase in caloric intake," the researchers reported. "Exercise . . . can be a useful treatment for weight reduction."

That's fine. But will exercise

Do you keep the frantic pace of the stress-filled business executive? If so, you might do well to get in step with these New York City executives who spend their lunch hour jogging through Central Park. A study of American wage earners showed that company executives are 7.7 times more likely to have a heart attack than coal miners and 6 times more likely than physicians.

5

Another Benefit—Quick Reaction Time

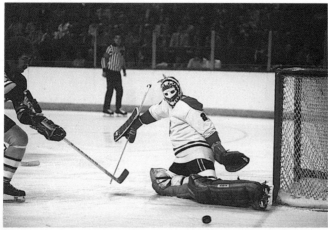

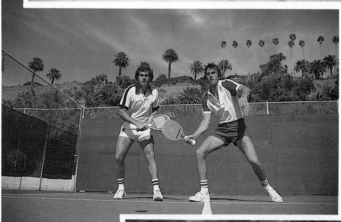

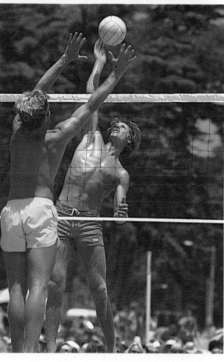

Aerobic activity can do more than keep your heart young and healthy. It can also keep your reactions sharp. Without exercise, your reaction time can slow down. Hockey, racquet games and volleyball are good reaction sports.

work for people who don't live in a hospital, people who have access to food that *they* prepare (or maybe just buy and binge on)? Again, the studies say yes. In fact, they say that dieting *without* exercise might be a waste of time.

In one experiment, researchers put 22 overweight women— "many of whom had failed at previous attempts to lose weight by dieting alone"—on an exercise and diet program. The women, according to the researchers, "were free to select their own method of dietary change," and most of them made "only moderate alterations of diet." But they altered their activity a lot. Four times a week for 17 weeks the women attended exercise classes. In two classes they walked and jogged for 20 minutes; in the other they did calisthenics and stretching for an hour. Did the program work?

After 17 weeks, the women had lost an average of 9 pounds. But they also gained something. There was an apparent increase in self-confidence in the group, and many of the women were very enthusiastic about the weight reduction program. (Can you say the same about the diets you've been on?) "They indicated that the . . . exercise approach gave them a feeling of accomplishment they had not experienced in previous attempts at dieting alone," said the researchers. "Many also noted that their increased physical work capacity enabled them to participate in and enjoy other forms of regular moderate and more vigorous exercise, which they had previously avoided."

In short, exercise changed their *lives,* not just the numbers on the scale. But it also changed their bodies in a way that dieting can't.

When you diet without exercising, says Gabe Mirkin, M.D., an expert in sports medicine and coauthor of *The Sportsmedicine Book*, you lose muscle as well as fat. But if you gain your weight back after the diet (and how many of us don't?), all of it will be in the form of fat. So you will have even more fat on your body than before you dieted, and because you now have less muscle you'll probably be more inactive and gain more weight. That's a vicious circle with a 40-inch waist.

When you diet *and* exercise (or

just exercise), you lose a lot of fat and gain a little muscle. The 22 women in the study, for instance, lost about 12 pounds of fat and gained about 3 pounds of muscle. That meant at the end of the program they were not only thinner, they were also *firmer.*

And healthier.

Overweight is a risk factor for a medical dictionary's worth of diseases. Stroke. Arthritis. Breast cancer. That list also includes diabetes, in which the body loses its ability to regulate blood sugar. In fact, diabetes and overweight (obesity) are so closely linked that one doctor dubbed the problem "diabesity." They also have a treatment in common. You guessed it. Exercise.

A SWEET SOLUTION

There are two kinds of diabetes and they have a generation gap. One is called juvenile-onset; the other, adult-onset. People with the first type, which usually develops in childhood, are shackled to injections of insulin, the hormone that controls blood sugar. If they miss a shot, they can go into a coma and die. In the second, which usually develops in middle age and hits millions of Americans, blood sugar control is also out of whack but not so badly as to require insulin shots. Badly enough, though, so that the extra sugar in the blood corrodes the circulation, leading to problems as serious as gangrene.

Exercise can't cure juvenile-onset diabetes, of course—it's too thorny a problem for that. (In fact, people who need insulin shots *must* consult with their doctor before starting an exercise program, because it could actually make their condition worse.) But it can help. Studies show, for instance, that kids need less insulin when they're at summer camp. And one experiment found that exercise lowers the stickiness of a juvenile-onset diabetic's blood to normal levels—a change that researchers think might stop a symptom called diabetic retinopathy, hemorrhages in the blood vessels of the eye that can cause blindness.

Adult-onset diabetes is a different story. Exercise can just about

Age Doesn't Matter—If You Exercise

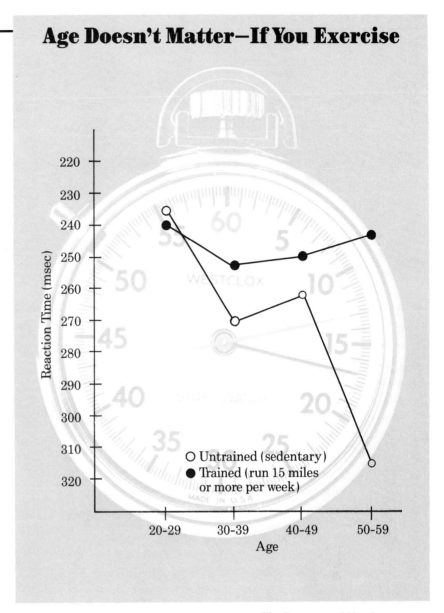

erase the disease. In one study, researchers put nine of these diabetics on an exercise program. After a few months, they measured the patients' glucose tolerance—the body's ability to handle blood sugar. It returned to nearly normal in eight of the patients, leading the researchers to recommend that exercise should be an "important treatment" in adult-onset diabetes. It should also be an important *preventive* measure.

Scientists at Yale University put six healthy but inactive men on an exercise program: 1 hour of vigorous exercise four times a week. After six weeks on the program, the men had a 30 percent increase in "tissue sensitivity" to insulin—it took less insulin to move excess blood sugar out of the circulation into storage. They also had a 50 percent increase

The Fountain of Youth just may be at your local track. At least that's what researchers at the San Diego State University found after testing 64 male and female volunteers, ranging in age from 23 to 59, for reaction time. Half the volunteers were serious runners, averaging 42 miles a week. The other half did no exercise at all. As the chart shows, researchers found that trained runners, *regardless* of age, experienced no average slowing of their reaction times. But reaction time got slower with age for the sedentary folks! The researchers concluded that a high state of cardiovascular training might be good for mental performance.

in the number of "cell receptors" for insulin, the tiny doors on cells that let the hormone in to do its work. Both these changes mean that the body's insulin manufacturer—the pancreas—had to do less work. And that's a plus, because adult-onset diabetes may start when the pancreas collapses from a lifetime of overtime (probably caused by eating too much sugar day after day). But the pancreas isn't the only organ that exercise helps. It's kind to your gallbladder, too.

HOW TO PREVENT GALLSTONES

The gallbladder is a cucumber-shaped sack that stores the bile manufactured by the liver and then relays it to your intestines, where it helps break down fat. The bile itself is a concoction of water, minerals, a couple of exotic chemicals—and cholesterol. The cholesterol was picked up by the liver (which actually puts this heart-hater to good use, such as the synthesis of hormones), and is just along for the ride. But it can become a nasty hitchhiker and knife the gallbladder—or at least get the surgeon to do it. When cholesterol in the bile clumps together, like snow-flakes being packed into a snowball, it forms a mass that doctors call a gallstone. When a gallstone becomes lodged in the delicate tubes and tissues of the gallbladder and causes lots of pain (and maybe costs you lots of money if it and your gallbladder have to be removed), you call it a . . . well, we can't print that.

But what causes cholesterol to form a stone? Some say it's a fatty diet. A doctor at the University of Cincinnati School of Medicine says a no-exercise lifestyle also has a lot to do with it.

He reports studies where scientists measured the "solubility" of cholesterol in the bile of people before and after they exercised—that is, whether or not the cholesterol would form a stone. In every case, exercise improved the solubility of cholesterol so that stones were less likely to form. "Lack of exercise should be considered an important factor in the [formation] of cholesterol gallstones," he says.

But while you don't want a rock in your gallbladder, you *do* want the minerals in your bones to stay there and keep them hard. Without exercise, that might not happen.

STRONGER MUSCLES, STRONGER BONES

The only skeletons most of us ever look at are the leering window decorations of Halloween. But if you could see your own, you might really be scared—because so much of it is missing it's more like a ghost! A typical 70-year-old woman, for example, has lost *30 percent* of her bone. Why was the cruel trick—called osteoporosis—played on her? Because she didn't treat herself to exercise.

The bones of athletes prove the point. A bone in the playing arm of a tennis pro can be 35 percent bigger than the same bone in his nonplaying

Asthmatics *Can* Exercise

Exercise and asthma don't mix, right? Not necessarily. Medical studies show that, contrary to popular opinion, certain types of exercise can actually help control asthma by reducing airway constriction. Activities that involve brief spurts of action, separated by rests, are less apt to cause asthma attacks than sports that require continuous exertion. So, what's ideal? Swimming, say some experts. Baseball, golf and even cycling—provided there are proper pauses—are also good.

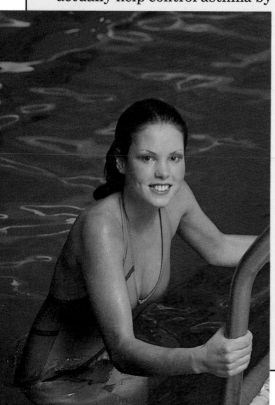

A Look at a Healthy Muscle

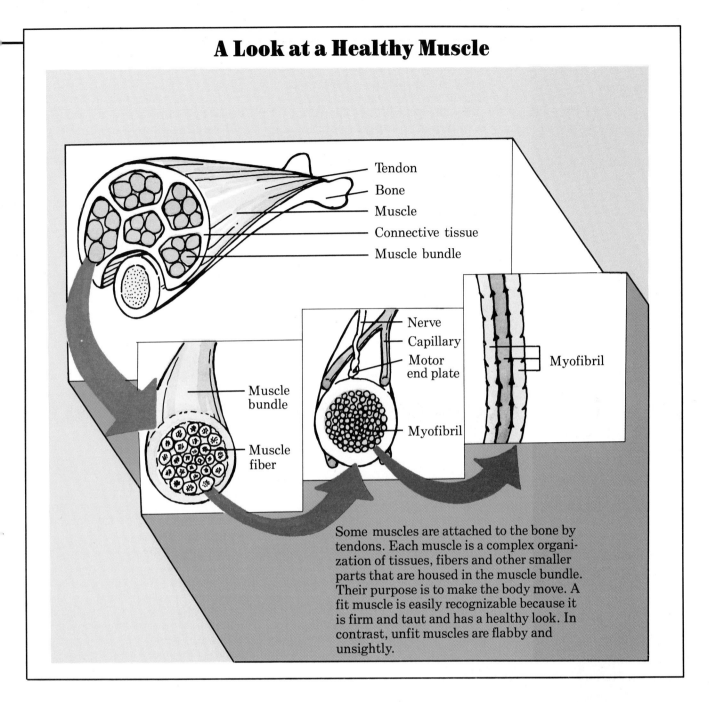

Tendon
Bone
Muscle
Connective tissue
Muscle bundle

Muscle bundle
Muscle fiber

Nerve
Capillary
Motor end plate
Myofibril

Myofibril

Some muscles are attached to the bone by tendons. Each muscle is a complex organization of tissues, fibers and other smaller parts that are housed in the muscle bundle. Their purpose is to make the body move. A fit muscle is easily recognizable because it is firm and taut and has a healthy look. In contrast, unfit muscles are flabby and unsightly.

arm. A baseball pitcher has more bone in his throwing arm. Bone is a living tissue, and like muscle it responds to stress by becoming stronger and larger. But you don't have to be a superstar to have super bones.

A team of doctors studied a group of 30 older women. Eighteen were nonexercisers and 12 were in an exercise program for three years. During that time, the inactive group lost 3.3 percent of the minerals in their bones, while the active group gained 2.3 percent. Also, the inactive group's bones thinned by 2.6 percent, while the active group's bones thickened by 1.7 percent.

Don't get the idea that older women are the only ones who have to worry about their bones. A study conducted by two physical education professors looked at students—45 men and 45 women between the ages of 20 and 25. They were asked about their activity levels and then ranked into three groups: high, moderate and low activity. When their bone density was measured, the researchers found that the high-activity group had denser bones than the moderate and low groups. "A physical activity lifestyle above the sedentary level is needed to . . . stave off the threat of osteoporosis in later years," said the researchers.

And since for hormonal reasons this disease does strike more women than men, they added that "young girls especially, as a safeguard against early onset of osteoporosis, must participate in vigorous physical activity during their growing years to generate maximal bone strength and density."

Or, as one doctor said about bone loss, "Prevention makes better sense than treatment." The same could be said about aging.

LOOK YOUNGER, FEEL YOUNGER

Prevent aging? What do we think exercise is, a time machine?

No, we agree with Andrew Ostrow, Ph.D., a professor at West Virginia University, when he says, "There is no proof that exercise can add years to your life." But aging doesn't just mean blowing out more candles on your birthday cake. It means change. Muscles changing to fat. Strength changing to weakness. Clarity changing to confusion. Most of us think these changes are the tax we owe Father Time. Dr. Ostrow thinks differently. "We have overestimated the effects of aging and underestimated the importance of remaining physically active."

Dr. Walter Bortz, an internist from Palo Alto, California, seconds the motion: "A review of biologic changes commonly attributed to the process of aging demonstrates the close similarity of most of these changes subsequent to a period of enforced physical inactivity." (In other words, if a person has to stay in bed for six weeks, at the end of the period his body is *years* older. It's atrophied from lack of use.) That similarity, he says, leads him to believe that "at least a portion of the changes that are commonly attributed to aging are in reality caused by disuse and are subject to correction." Now that's exciting news! What kind of correction does Dr. Bortz have in mind? "Exercise."

And other doctors have proved that it works.

A doctor from the University of Wisconsin Medical School studied 28 people between the ages of 62 and 85.

They were in an exercise program for three months. At the end of that time, their fitness levels were about the same as those of an inactive 30-year-old.

In another study at the University of Wisconsin, a group of 40 people between the ages of 65 and 88 improved their joint flexibility—their range of motion—between 8 and 48 percent after three months of exercise.

In a study of two women "masters" swimmers (older people who race against others their age), researchers found their levels of body fat were the same as those of average women 19 to 25 years old. "Regular training may delay the accumulation of excess fat that accompanies inactivity during aging," said the researchers.

Scientists have also found that exercise restores lung power, endurance and strength. So while it's true you can't cheat Father Time, at least you can get a refund.

AVOID THOSE NAGGING NUISANCES

The health problems we've talked about so far—like heart disease, bone loss or diabetes—are some of life's 12-inch guns. They can sink you for good. But what about the potshots— problems like insomnia, headache or colds? Can exercise do anything about them? Take off your helmet and relax while we review some of the clauses in the peace treaty.

Allergy. A study reported in the *Journal of Allergy* showed that exercise can open the swollen nasal passages of a person with hay fever. In seven people tested, all had an increase in their airway passages after exercising.

Colds and Flu. A team of researchers from Purdue University and the University of Arizona examined the twin effects of exercise and vitamin supplements on immunity, with exciting results. "We found that vitamins C and E were important in improving immune function, but exercise strongly *augmented* these effects," they reported. "The improvement is really a significant one, too."

The researchers subjected a group of volunteers to a four-month regimen of vitamins C and E, or a 1½-hour workout three times a week, or both vitamins and workouts, or neither one. Throughout the study period, they kept tabs on their subjects' immunological strength by measuring T-cells (infection fighters) in their blood.

"There was a significant effect of vitamin supplementation with the high-fit group compared to the low-fit group in terms of increase in percent of T-cells," they reported. "However, the high-fit group had higher mitogenesis (T-cell production) regardless of supplementation. Apparently both physical conditioning and high intake of vitamins can stimulate cellular immune functions in adults."

Headaches. Researchers at the University of Wisconsin have used exercise to treat migraine headaches, with remarkable success. Nine sedentary people who were regularly visited by migraines carefully recorded the frequency and intensity of their headaches—but didn't exercise—for the first five weeks of the study. For the following ten weeks they walked or ran three days a week for at least 30 minutes.

And when they finished this regimen, the nine subjects reported their headaches were showing up 50 percent less often. When they *did* show up, they were slightly less severe than before the training program began.

Insomnia. A team of psychologists tested eight people, four who were fit and four who were out of shape. They found that the fit people had more "slow-wave sleep"—the stages of sleep that are more restorative and refreshing.

Skin Problems. A team of Finnish researchers found that people who exercise regularly may have thicker, stronger skin. The researchers compared 50 runners and cross-country skiers, who trained about 30 miles a week, with 50 healthy but untrained men. They found that the trained men's skin was thicker and more flexible. The researchers also theorize that exercise may slow down the aging of skin.

HIGH-ENERGY LIVING

So far we've talked about 50 percent of you: your body. What about your mind? Well, exercise doesn't do things by halves. It uplifts your spirits along with those more physical sags.

In a study at Duke University Medical Center, researchers asked 16

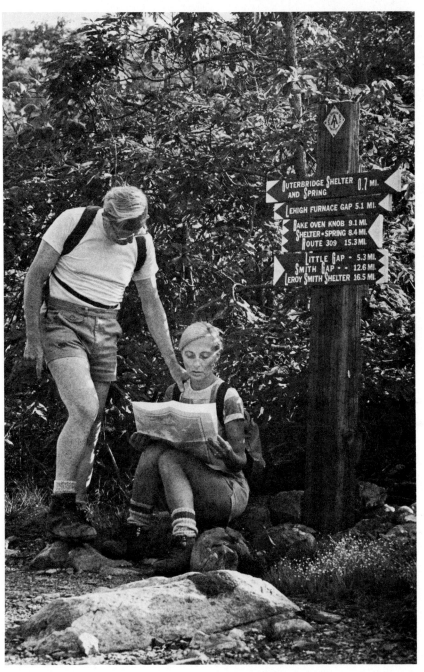

It's easy to measure the benefits exercise has on the heart in terms of our physical well-being, but there's another benefit to the heart that's a little harder to measure. That's the bond it can make between families and friends who share their exercise experiences together.

healthy, middle-aged volunteers to participate in a ten-week program of regular walking or jogging. A second group maintained their inactive lifestyles. Before and after the experiment, both groups took psychological tests designed to measure their levels of anxiety, depression, vigor and fatigue.

At the end of the experiment, the researchers found that 61 percent of the exercisers felt an enhanced sense of personal achievement, compared to only 27 percent of the inactive group. The exercise group also experienced reductions in anxiety, felt more vigor and less tension, depression and fatigue than their sedentary counterparts.

"In virtually every comparison," said the researchers, "the exercise group tended to change in the desired direction, whereas the inactive group remained the same or actually got worse . . . our data suggests that basically healthy, well-adjusted people can increase their sense of well-being compared to healthy people who do not exercise."

A lot of us aren't "well adjusted" all the time. In fact, studies show that *most* of us will sooner or later suffer from a bout of depression. We'll feel tired, sad or apathetic. We won't have any appetite for food or sex. And physical problems—like back pain or headache—will hang like parasites on our mental state.

John Greist, M.D., a psychiatrist and a professor at the University of Wisconsin, has studied the effect of running on depression. Dr. Greist is a runner himself, and he decided to try it on his patients after he noticed that if he felt irritable or low when he started to jog, by the end of the run he usually felt great.

As a scientist, Dr. Greist had to *prove* that running was at least as good as psychotherapy before recommending it to his patients. So he divided depressed patients—15 women and 13 men, aged 18 to 30—into three groups. One group ran. One group had time-limited psychotherapy, which means that the date the treatment ends is specified ahead of time. One group had time-unlimited psychotherapy. Depression levels on a scale of 1 to 4 were measured before, during and at the end of the study (1 meant a little depressed; 2, moderately; 3, quite a bit; 4, extremely). The results?

The patients who had time-limited psychotherapy scored an average of just below 1 on the depression scale. The patients in time-unlimited therapy averaged just below 2. The patients who ran, however, averaged just above *zero*—not at all depressed.

Dr. Greist isn't the only one who has conducted studies like this. Robert Brown, M.D., Ph.D., a psychiatrist and a professor at the University of Virginia, studied 101 depressed college students. He divided them into two groups, one that exercised regularly and one that didn't.

"Jogging five days a week for a ten-week period was associated with significant reductions in depression scores," says Dr. Brown. "Similar patterns were exhibited by those who jogged only three days a week for the same period. The subjects who did not exercise during the same interval had virtually unchanged scores."

How-to books. Records. State-of-the-art equipment. Health clubs. You needn't look far to realize that the opportunity to enhance our lives through fitness is literally at our fingertips.

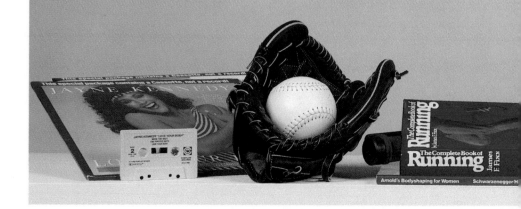

Exercise Changed Their Lives

"I had an irregular heartbeat till I began running," Joan Bordow from Richmond, California, says. "My body and whole sense of self were transformed from weak to strong. Now I'm 39, a writer and feel great."

Lawyer Sandra Glanz Porter of Dallas, Texas, started running during college out of frustration and also for personal achievement. "Running gives me energy. I need it and it gives me a whole new day, every day."

Steve Hillinger, a holistic healing practitioner from Portland, Oregon, went through a major life awakening and says, "The ritual of exercise played a big role for me as a part of the metaphor of health through diet, exercise and rest."

"I'm studying opera and found that yoga taught me to let go in mind and body. I couldn't do what I'm doing without it," says 30-year-old Jeff Robinson of New York City.

"I began a serious program of Nautilus and running about 3 years ago as a release. I'd die without it," claims Sam Hess, former manager of a retail office building in Philadelphia.

Dr. Brown also gave the depressed students "adjective checklists" that described their emotional states. Among the depressed subjects who jogged, according to Dr. Brown, negative states of anger/hostility, fatigue/inertia and tenseness/anxiety decreased. Positive states of cheerfulness and energy increased.

Energy. Isn't that what life is all about? The energy to give special attention to your family and friends. The energy to take up new interests and see new places. The energy to succeed at work without feeling worn down. Exercise is a perfect way to get that energy, to recharge yourself with happiness and health. And isn't it great knowing that *you* control the switch?

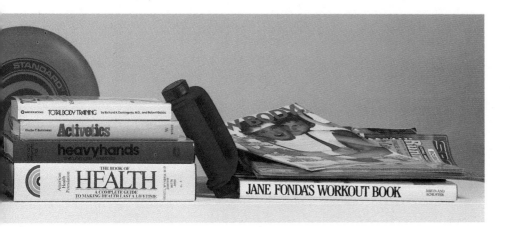

2

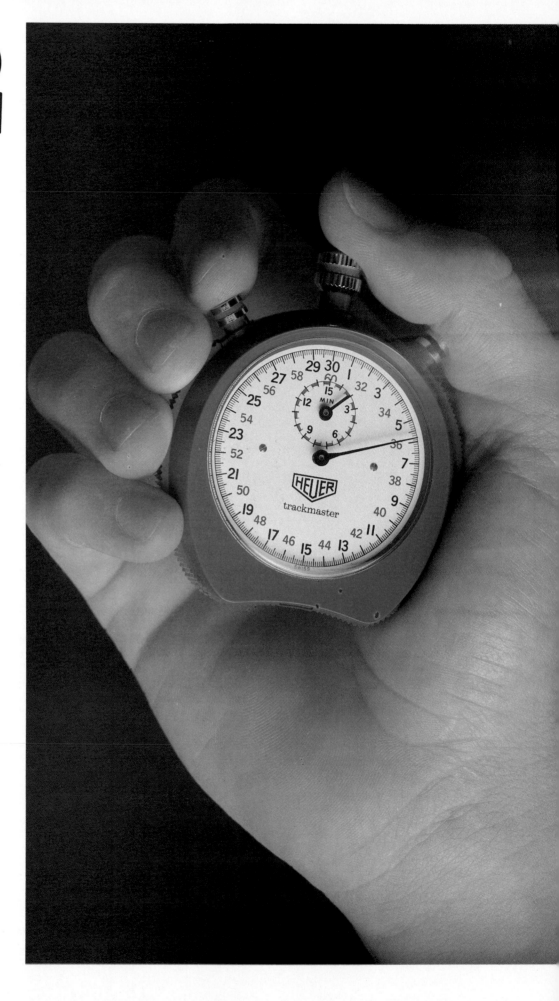

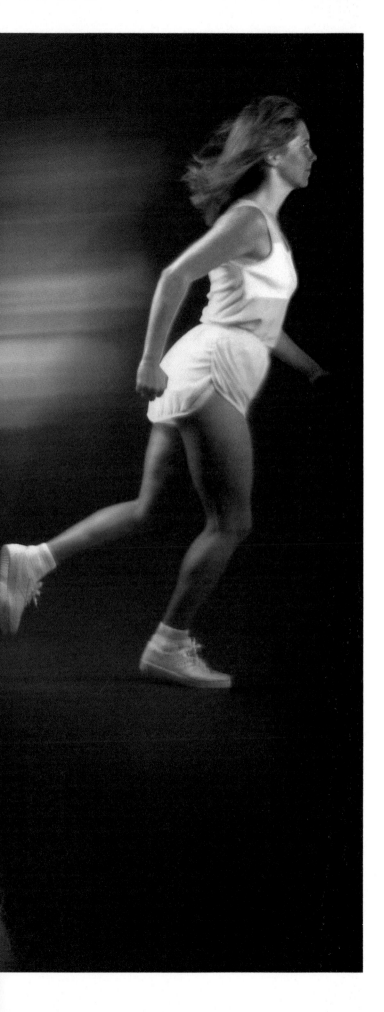

Let's Get Motivated

Getting a body conditioning program off to a sure start calls for a bit of mind conditioning.

H ere's a scenario you may know too well. The winter's been a dreary one and the first warm day of spring has you hankering for the not-too-distant days when you can stretch out on the warm and sunny beach. You can even visualize yourself sunning lazily on the sand, your svelte body exuding vigor and sensuality. So you check the real corpus delicti in the mirror: svelte it ain't. You hold your breath as you try to squeeze into last year's bathing suit. Bad news: It looks—and feels—two sizes too small. The accumulated results of winter sloth hang around your waist. What's a body to do?

Exercise, you say. Tone up the old flabby muscles while cutting back on calories. Make the visualization a reality. And so you start a new exercise regimen with a vengeance. After all, bathing suit season isn't all that far away.

Day one is tough, but you manage. Day two hurts because you overdid day one. On day three you oversleep, so forget the morning workout. Exercise after work somehow falls by the wayside, too. Day four dawns on what little resolve you have left, and that's challenged at lunchtime by hunger pangs and the seductive aroma coming from the nearby pizzeria. Your complete breakdown is just 30 steps and one bite away. And you succumb! With that first delicious morsel comes the haunting refrain of an exercise program gone awry: "So what's exercise going to do for me now that I ate all that heavy food?" you reason with yourself. "Besides, my muscles are still sore from the beginning of the week. And the weekend's just about here anyway. I guess I'll just start all over again on Monday."

Sound familiar? The cycle of exercise and regression is so prevalent that some people think it's as inevitable as the tides. And they're half right. Some approaches to exercise are doomed to failure before the sneakers touch the ground. Others, however, give you far better odds of succeeding. They increase your chances of starting off on the right foot, enjoying the regimen and staying with it for the long haul.

So what's the big success secret? No big secret. What you find when you sift through the winning approaches are a few get-in-shape principles that fitness experts have been using for years.

Take It Easy. The idea is *not* to whip yourself into shape. That hurts. The point is to *ease* yourself into fitness. If you try to break world records right at the start, you're going to injure yourself—and get very discouraged awfully fast.

Lowell Scott Weil, D.P.M., a podiatrist from Des Plaines, Illinois, suggests that our bodies may know more about slow-and-easy fitness than we do. "Injuries often occur because people do not listen to the messages their own bodies send them. They hear that exercise is painful, so when it begins to hurt, they push harder, when maybe they should stop. They forget that exercise involves regular but *moderate* demands placed on the body and its systems."

For a lot of people, however, taking it easy is not so easy. That's why so many exercise specialists talk about planning.

Charles Kuntzleman, Ed.D., a national consultant to the YMCA, is one of them. He says you should plan an attainable exercise quota for your first month and promise yourself a reward for reaching that short-term goal. You should be absolutely sure you can handle the quota—and up the ante only when you're sure you're ready for a tougher challenge. Forget about long-range goals, says Dr. Kuntzleman: "They can often make you feel like a failure or discourage you."

To help you stick with your game plan, he recommends keeping an exercise diary. It can help you monitor your progress and keep reminding you how well you're doing.

Be Realistic about Results. Sometimes your biggest stumbling block to effective exercise is not the clock, the weather or your reluctant sinews. It's your head. An unrealistic notion can stop you as quickly as a broken leg.

And the champion pie-in-the-sky idea is that exercise gives instant results without the slightest discomfort. Advertisements promise weight loss at the rate of 10 pounds a week and big muscles in seven days. Instantaneous fitness is the fashion, and sedentary people are eager to be in vogue. Disappointment is in the air.

Those who stick with an exercise routine are usually the ones who've faced the facts. Exercise does produce impressive results, but it's never going to be as effortless as swaying in the hammock.

"Learn to expect that exercise involves a workout that is not totally easy," says Dr. Kuntzleman. "If you're bored the first mile, or it seems rough when you start out, tell yourself it gets better and work at it.

Get Off Your "Can't"!

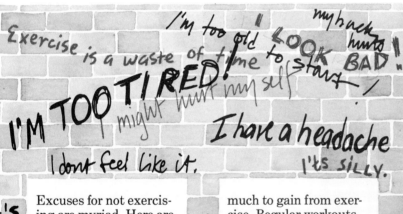

Excuses for not exercising are myriad. Here are a few all-time favorites, and the reasons why they just aren't valid.

Exercise isn't safe. Medical evidence suggests that exercising is safer than not exercising. People who get hurt are usually trying to do too much too fast.

I'm too old. Nobody's too old. Studies show that exercise is for all ages.

I have too much to do. Busy people have much to gain from exercise. Regular workouts increase stamina and sharpen concentration, boosting productivity.

The weather's bad. So go around it. Wear appropriate clothes and step outdoors anyway. Or, work out in a gym or spa. Any program can be modified for indoor exertion.

I have arthritis. Proper exercise (water exercise is particularly helpful) can soothe sore muscles and joints.

You can expect some stiffness and soreness at first, but that can actually help you psychologically. It shows that exercise is developing your body."

Confront the Time Problem. Come to terms with the almighty clock—the bane of so many exercise schedules—and you greatly enhance your chances of staying with your regimen. Coming to terms means recognizing that exercise time is not the rarity that some people think it is. Joe Henderson, author of *Jog, Run, Race*, thinks that some people have an exaggerated idea of how much time a good workout takes. About 30 minutes a day is all you need, he says.

"Anybody who cannot squeeze a half hour out of the day is not organizing his day well," he explains. "That person needs to take inventory of his time. Maybe he can shorten lunch, or not watch a TV show at night. But there is some place during the day when 30 minutes can be found."

Fitness expert Tom Griffin, M.D., author of *Feeling Good for Life*, agrees. He points out that squeezing in an exercise routine is a cinch—once you get your priorities straight.

"Pay yourself first," he says, "Instead of 'spending' the 24 hours of each day in work, sleep, eating, entertainment, family, etc., allot 30 minutes to yourself first—then divide the remainder. You'll have plenty of time left to do all the other things."

For many people, that golden half hour comes in the morning before work, at lunchtime or in the evening before dinner. But there are exceptions galore, and you'll have to decide if you're one of them. Or, rather, your body will decide. For one thing, you can't ignore its biological clock. If the clock says you're a morning person, you exercise in the morning. If it says night, then night it is. But you *don't* work out when your body sends you signals of fatigue, fever or hunger. Working out when you're feverish or dead tired is begging for calamity. And exercising when you haven't eaten for 12 hours (like before your morning glass of juice) can leave you out of breath and out of steam before your workout is over.

Go for Health. Some people exercise to avoid ill health; others exercise to get to higher levels of good health. Which group is more likely to ride their program the distance and enjoy the trip?

The good-health crowd, of course. They're going for the carrot on the stick—ever loftier planes of wellness. The other bunch is just trying to stay out of harm's way.

"It's difficult for people to get motivated by the idea that exercise helps prevent physical problems," says Dr. Griffin. "It's much easier to get excited about the fact that exercise helps you live longer and makes you feel great."

So go for the carrot, and the rest will take care of itself.

Remember the Fun Factor. How long are you likely to stay committed to an exercise regimen that's about as pleasurable as Chinese water torture?

About a minute, probably. Yet every day people try to throw themselves at a workout they hate.

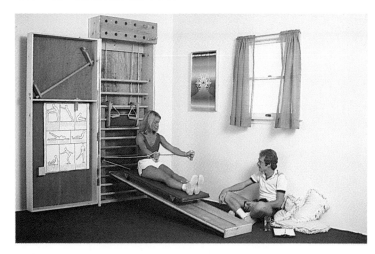

They overlook the pleasure principle of exercise: A regimen must be fun—or it soon becomes no regimen at all.

Says Dr. Griffin, "Fun is critical in any exercise program. Where or when you exercise may be important. But neither variable is as crucial as whether you're having a good time. You have to consider an exercise's potential for pleasure." Some people have trouble starting an exercise routine because to them exercise is anything but fun.

"Part of the inertia problem," says Jim Fixx, author of *The Complete Book of Running*, "is that too many of us were taught to look on exercise as punishment, or at the very least as an activity that isn't notably pleasurable."

The solution is a bit of mental reprogramming. You convince yourself that you were all wrong about exercise—by starting with a regimen you can't possibly dislike. Dorothy Harris, Ph.D., an internationally known sports physiologist from Pennsylvania State University, suggests people can make sure exercise is fun by "pursuing activities that are fairly easily learned. That's why racquetball is good. It's an easier sport to play than tennis or squash."

Make a Commitment. If you take promises seriously, says Fixx, making a commitment may be all you need to ensure your long-term devotion to an exercise program. A simple pledge to yourself to work out at a given hour for a given length of time may be motivation enough.

And such a commitment is a good idea even if you're not so good at keeping promises to yourself. The pledge—whether shaky or as solid as stone—will be one more barrier to giving up.

That pledge will become particularly important when temptation starts to lure you toward that corner

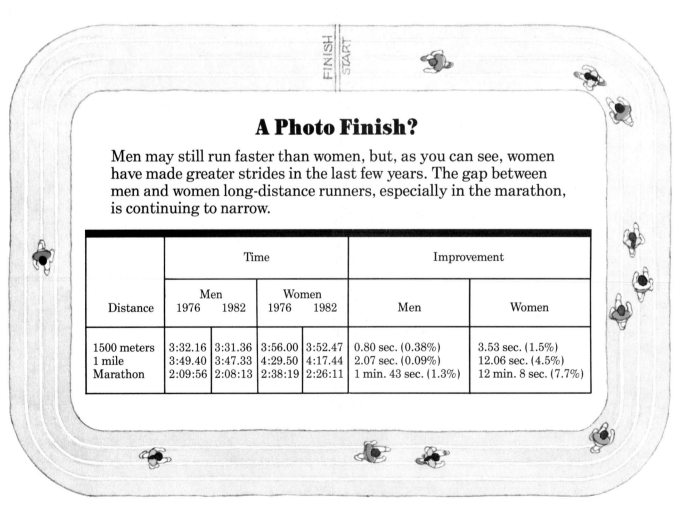

A Photo Finish?

Men may still run faster than women, but, as you can see, women have made greater strides in the last few years. The gap between men and women long-distance runners, especially in the marathon, is continuing to narrow.

Distance	Time				Improvement	
	Men		Women		Men	Women
	1976	1982	1976	1982		
1500 meters	3:32.16	3:31.36	3:56.00	3:52.47	0.80 sec. (0.38%)	3.53 sec. (1.5%)
1 mile	3:49.40	3:47.33	4:29.50	4:17.44	2.07 sec. (0.09%)	12.06 sec. (4.5%)
Marathon	2:09:56	2:08:13	2:38:19	2:26:11	1 min. 43 sec. (1.3%)	12 min. 8 sec. (7.7%)

The Benefits of Exercise

Exercise	Warm-Up	Aerobic Fitness	Flexibility	Toning	Strength	Cool-Down
Aerobic dancing	●	●●●		●●●		●
Aqua aerobics	●●	●●●	●●●	●		●●●
Bench press				●	●●●	
Cross-country skiing	●	●●●				●●
Curl				●●	●●●	
Cycling	●●	●●●		●●●		●●
Dumbbell fly			●●	●●	●●●	
Ice skating		●●●		●●		●
Jogging/running	●	●●●		●		●
Martial arts	●●●		●●●	●●●	●	●●●
Overhead press				●●	●●●	
Pushups				●	●●	
Racquetball		●●●		●●		●
Rowing	●	●●●		●●●		●●
Side lean	●●●		●●●			●●●
Squat				●●	●●	
Squat thrust	●	●●		●●		●
Standing toe touch			●●●			●●●
Walking	●●●	●		●		●●●
Yoga			●●●	●●		●●●

KEY:
○ beginner
○ intermediate
● advanced

The benefits you derive from individual exercises will change as you progress through your fitness program. For example, the body toning you may notice as you progress as an ice skater will taper off once you get in the advanced league. At this point, the only thing you'll be improving is your aerobic fitness. Also, some exercises are more useful as warm-ups and cool-downs to those who are fit than to the not-so-fit. This chart should give you an idea of the benefits you'll reap from some of the more popular exercises, depending on your level of fitness.

pizzeria. It doesn't take a genius to realize that exercise takes on an extra dimension of importance during times of personal gluttony. Exercise burns up a lot of calories—even walking is a whole lot better than just sitting around. So, if you give in to temptation and go on an eating binge, it's no time to give up on exercise! When you become a regular exerciser and honor your commitment, too many calories today will instinctively lead you to an even harder workout tomorrow.

Excuse-Proof Your Program. The day you begin working out is the day you'll suddenly become aware of a ton of obstacles. Getting up an hour earlier in the morning is harder than

you thought. It's too dark in the evening to walk or jog outdoors. You don't like exercising alone. If these excuses don't occur to you, others will.

You might as well tackle them head on or your exercise program will be in jeopardy from day one. Sit down and make a list of the things you think will interfere with your regimen, then devise solutions for each problem.

You may have to go to bed an hour earlier to relieve that morning droop. Or use an indoor jogging track. Or find a friend who's willing to exercise with you.

"Getting involved with other people is critical," says Dr. Harris. "It takes a very disciplined person to

The All-Weather Runner

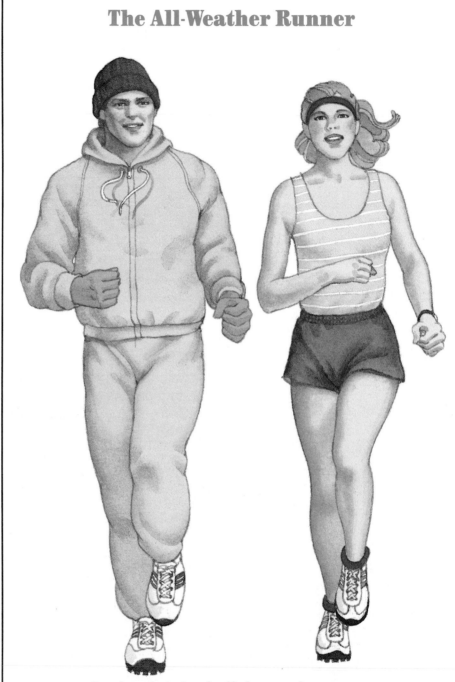

Outdoor jogging buffs have to be more creative in their dress than those who are content to pound the track indoors. In cold weather a few layers of lightweight clothing are all you'll ever need as long as you cover your extremities. A cap is a must—it keeps your body heat from escaping. Gloves keep frostbite away. In summer, your biggest fear is heatstroke. Lightweight and airy togs are musts.

exercise entirely on his or her own. Togetherness is why weight reduction groups, Alcoholics Anonymous and Gamblers Anonymous work so well. It keeps you motivated. Find someone comparable to your level of fitness, with similar aspirations, to exercise with."

Starting is always the hardest part. But you *can* make it easy on yourself, so that beginning again every day doesn't require such mammoth force of will. "Think through your daily routine, and see where you can incorporate exercise," says Dr. Harris. "Walk instead of ride, climb stairs instead of using the elevator, do stretches while you talk on the telephone." If you have the choice every morning of a pleasant hour's walk to work or an awful half hour on the subway, choose the walk.

Your particular solutions don't matter nearly as much as your willingness to take on the problems before they become insurmountable.

EXERCISE IS FOR EVERYONE

Actually, when you come right down to it, it's pretty hard to find a reason—a really good reason—for not exercising. *Everyone* can—and should—exercise.

Sex is certainly no excuse. Sure, in many tests of physical fitness males and females do show some basic differences, but these are a consequence of anatomical and physiological differences. Females adapt to training just as well as men.

Look at the current sports rosters. Women are now involved in virtually all sports and fitness activities and are even entering into areas such as weight training that used to be solely male preserves. There is even some evidence that women may be better suited for endurance training than men.

Age is irrelevant, too. Seven-year-olds and septuagenarians run marathons, although some doctors would not recommend such extreme workouts for children, because they believe that the shock from running can be harmful to growing bones and joints.

But then again, it's usually not children who have a problem motiva-

ting themselves to get out and exercise. It's adults. The common refrains of "I'm getting too old" or "I haven't moved a muscle in 20 years" are simply poor excuses to ignore exercise. As we've already pointed out in chapter 1, exercise can actually help *reverse* the signs of aging. And you don't have to become a hard-nosed devotee to make it work in your favor, either. Michael L. Pollock, Ph.D., of the Institute for

Prevent Sore Muscles

Sore muscles are the plague of many exercisers, particularly beginners. But the soreness can be minimized with special exercises. The ones shown here are best done with a partner. (1) Lie on your stomach and raise your legs as your partner applies downward resistance; (2) Lie on your stomach with your knees flexed and feet together and pull your feet apart as your partner applies resistance; (3) Do half-squats and/or stride out with one leg and then the other; (4) Do half sit-ups with your partner holding your feet.

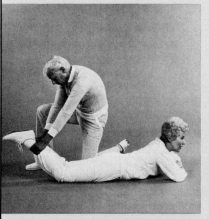
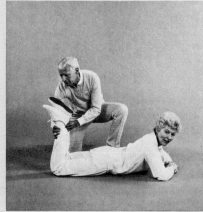
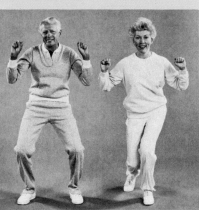
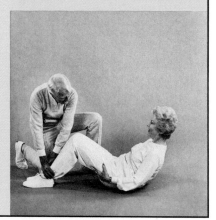

Aerobics Research in Dallas, studied the effects of training for 30 minutes a day three times a week on 22 sedentary men between the ages of 49 and 65. He found that regimen sufficient to make significant increases in their fitness levels.

THE SKY'S THE LIMIT

There seems to be no limit to what the body can do if the spirit is willing. Although there are physical problems that may affect the *type* of exercise you choose—weak knees or ankles, hip problems, obesity—an appropriate exercise program can be designed around most problems.

Special conditions like pregnancy, back problems, diabetes and arthritis can also impose certain limitations. But people with these conditions can participate in a regular exercise routine—and enjoy it, too. We'll get into that more in chapter 7.

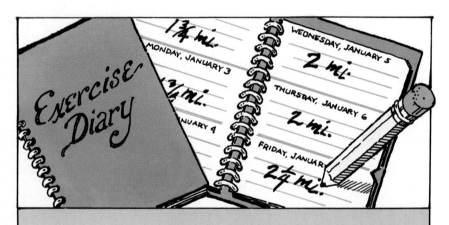

Athletes have been keeping journals for as long as there've been sports; they use them to record past feats and future goals. So why not take after the pros and start your own diary? For example, if you are a runner, a diary can show daily distances, times, mood swings, diet, exercise problems and how well you cope with temperature and humidity. Use it to record aches and pains. If you're a more-than-one exercise type, a wall calendar is handy for measuring the progress of one form of exercise against the others. Your diary can be your training partner, a good friend and, most of all, a valuable gauge of your health.

CHOOSING AN EXERCISE

The best exercise is one that strengthens the heart and respiratory system. But exercise should also improve muscular strength and increase flexibility. Unfortunately, no single exercise can really accomplish all three goals.

Running, for example, is very good for the heart and lungs and the muscles of the legs, but it does little for upper body strength. Cycling is much like running. A tennis or racquetball match is valuable for aerobic exercise only if the skill level of both players is equal.

Sports such as weight lifting, football, wrestling, hockey, volleyball, basketball and gymnastics don't benefit the heart nearly as much as long-distance running, rowing, swimming and cross-country skiing do. In fact, only cross-country skiing and swimming are considered all-around exercises.

The best plan is to pick a primary method of exercise that is aerobic and supplement it from time to time with strength and flexibility exercise routines. Ideally, an exercise program includes:

- A warm-up period of 5 to 10 minutes of exercises designed to build up body heat and increase circulation and respiration. This protects muscles and joints from strain by reducing their resistance to movement. Stretching and calisthenic exercises serve this purpose.
- An endurance exercise that lasts from 20 to 30 minutes. Running, swimming or cycling is ideal.
- A tapering-off or cooling-down period of 5 to 10 minutes that includes exercises similar to those used in the warm-up, plus some deep breathing.

REAP THE BIG REWARDS

Of course, all this hard work has one primary goal—a better-looking and better-feeling you. You may eventually want to lose 30 pounds, do 100 sit-ups or run 10 miles, but it's important to understand that it will take time and effort to reach that goal.

The success of any exercise program is based on the progress made. The first few workouts won't bring about any immediate results, but in a couple of weeks you should find a noticeable difference both physically and mentally, and the soreness that was natural after your initial workouts will no longer be a problem. Not only will you find you have new strength and endurance and feel less fatigue, you also should have more energy, have lost some weight and even be sleeping better. This progress will continue as long as you continue to exercise, and it will keep you highly motivated.

You want this invigorating process to be a controlled one. You want real progress, but you want to neither overdo nor underdo.

A good rule of thumb is to work from plateau to plateau: Start off at a low level of exertion, work at it until it's easy for you, then move up to a higher stage. You can keep climbing or stay at a comfortable level.

As you move to a higher step, you should find yourself straining, struggling to get to the new plateau. That's called the "training effect," and it's just what's supposed to happen when you're going toward higher fitness.

The best rewards of all are the changes in your body and mind. Make the effort to actively notice them. Look for things on a daily basis. Notice your clothes fitting more loosely. (You may not notice changes on the scale, however, because muscle tissue weighs more than stored fat, even though it takes up less space.)

As your endurance builds, so will your enthusiasm. And, sure enough, the day will come when you discover that you like exercise after all.

The Warning Signs of Trouble

Exercise can be taxing on the body. For example, neglecting to warm up and cool down before and after exercising, or exercising too much, can be harmful to your health. A smart exerciser will be aware of the warning signs of trouble.

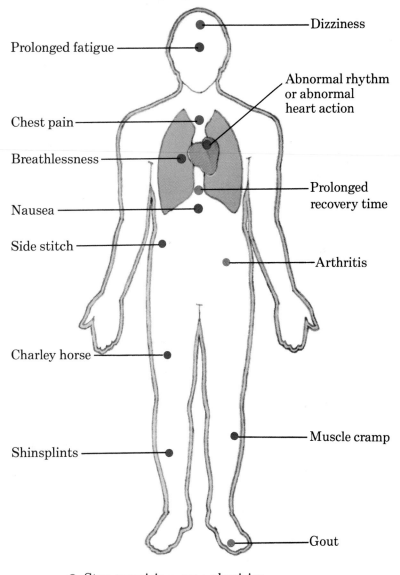

- ● Stop exercising; see a physician.
- ● Exercise more slowly. If condition persists, see a physician.
- ● Usually can be remedied on your own.

3

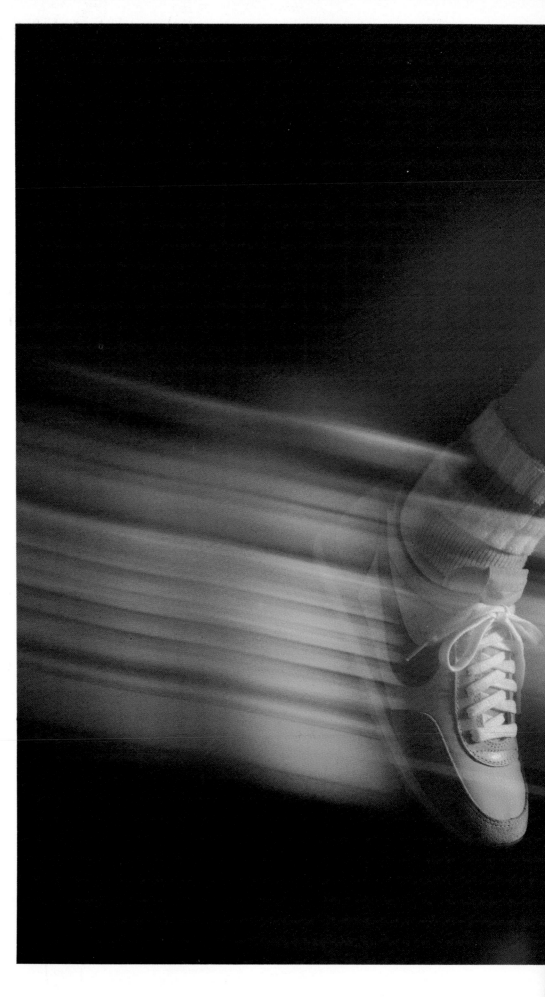

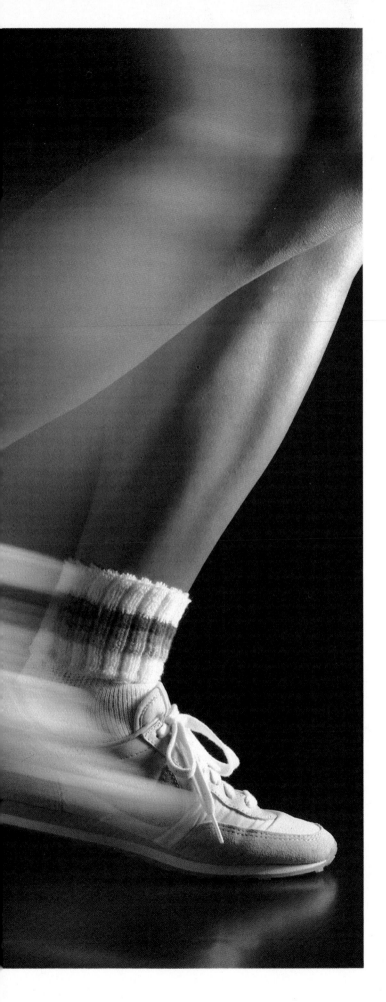

Aerobics: The All-Purpose Conditioner

There's nothing more vital to a fulfilling life than heart-pumping exercise.

United States Marines are in a foreign land; a volatile national election campaign makes assassins' targets out of political and spiritual leaders; young men are deserting the military.

The year is 1968.

And tucked quietly amidst all this upheaval and turmoil is the publication of a little book by a young military doctor, a book about exercise that calls for a revolution—an "aerobic revolution"—and for a healthier America.

These days, when Kenneth H. Cooper, M.D., opens his Dallas morning newspaper, it looks like the same old crazy world. But now, when he gazes out his window, Dr. Cooper can see more people than ever before running for health and fitness. And he can't get through the day without having the word "aerobic"—a term he made a household word as a result of his book *Aerobics*—jump out at him from book jackets, record covers, billboards and TV.

It seems that just about everyone you talk to these days is "into" aerobics—from the corner grocery store clerk to Jane Fonda. It's a term now so widely used that even those who refuse to exercise can't avoid it. To most people, though, aerobics simply means exercise. This definition isn't far off the mark. But aerobics is more than plain exercise. To be aerobic, an exercise must place a reasonable amount of stress on your heart and lungs. It must get you huffing and puffing—without stopping—for a good 30 minutes.

Of course, this extra exertion is not without its rewards. Aerobic exercise, better than anything else, gets you in shape. It gives you endurance. Your heart and blood vessels can more efficiently

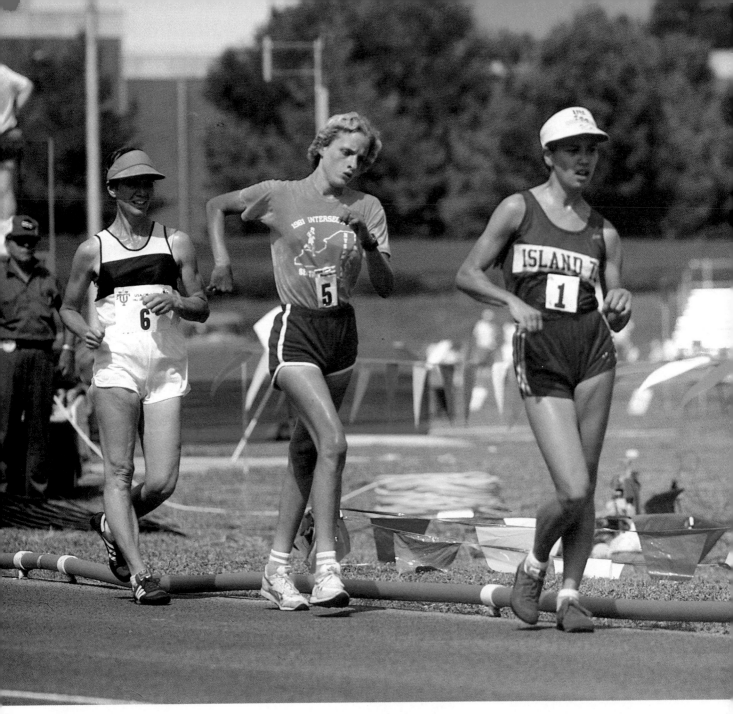

There are racers and there are walkers. And there are race-walkers. A breed of competitor all their own, race-walkers can often be spotted stride by stride with runners in marathon races. Some believe that the waddle-like, stiff stride that must be maintained is more grueling than running. Race-walking is even an Olympic event.

transport oxygen to the muscle cells, process the oxygen in those cells and carry off the waste. The rewards of such good cardiovascular fitness can be felt in every part of your body. You tire less easily, you get that sense of exuberant well-being that comes from good health and you decrease your chances of dying of a heart attack.

So, how do you achieve this marvelous state? With repetitive, rhythmic exercise. One that makes use of your body's large muscles. One that gets your heart beating faster — significantly faster — so it can "idle" much slower when you're idle yourself.

A friendly tennis game won't do it — too many pauses. The same goes for lifting weights, no matter how heavy. Cycling's good if it makes you breathe hot and heavy, and if you don't spend half your time coasting. Jogging is dandy — no matter how slowly you go.

PULSE RATE — GET IT LOW

As we said, the end-all of aerobic conditioning is a slower heartbeat. Another way of describing this is to say that you have a lower resting

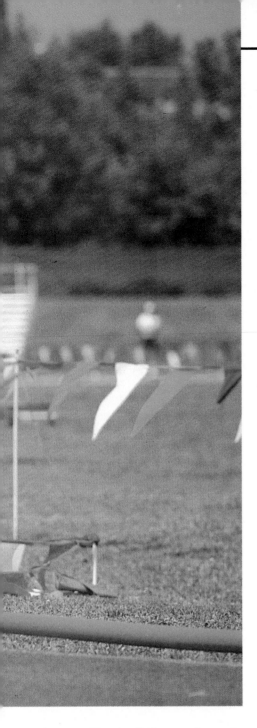

2 minutes) had resting heart rates of around 51 beats per minute. By contrast, those with marathon times of 6 to 6½ hours and 5.4 hours of weekly training had resting pulses of 67.6 beats per minute.

The reason that a low resting pulse rate is important—besides indicating that the heart is more efficiently pumping blood through the body—is that it shows the heart's ability to handle the enormous strain on the system produced by intense physical activity, high emotions and mental stress. Sometimes these factors can raise heart rates to as much as 200 beats per minute. And, as the researchers pointed out, if we consider 180 beats as a safe upper limit, then a resting rate of 90 can only double in emergencies before going over the safe limit—whereas a rate of 60 can triple. In other words, with a low resting pulse, your heart can better meet stress on its own terms without blowing your fuse. "We suggest," wrote the researchers, "that sudden deaths in sport, in saunas or after stress are more likely in people with higher resting pulse rates."

Researchers recommend raising the pulse rate during exercise to at least 70 or 80 percent of maximum. But how do you find 70 or 80 percent of your maximum? Simply use the number 220 as your absolute maximum pulse rate and then subtract your age from 220 to arrive at your age-adjusted maximum. For example, a 30-year-old would have an age-adjusted maximum of 190; 70 percent of that would be 133 beats per minute. However, it's important to keep in mind that none of this will do you any good unless you keep your pulse rate up for a good 30 minutes. And you should plan on exercising at that level *at least* three times a week.

Any of the exercises in this chapter are capable of getting you into aerobic condition. Pick one you like; that way, you'll probably stick with it. A healthier heart may be your reward.

pulse rate. But is all that work worth it? Just how important is it to have a low resting pulse rate? Well, it could be critical.

The lower the beat of your pulse (up to a point, of course; zero is a tad on the low side), the more prepared you are to accommodate physical and mental stresses and the more likely you are to stay healthy and live longer. Low resting pulse rate is linked directly to physical fitness. When British researchers looked at a number of marathon runners, they found that one group that spent 8.7 hours a week in training (and finished the marathon in under 3 hours,

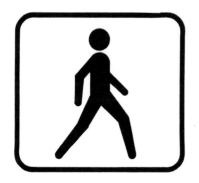

Walking

Experts agree: Walking is the single best type of exercise for millions of people who want to firm up, tone up and rev up.

The secret to turning a daily stroll into a meaningful form of exercise is to pick up the pace. The surprise that's in store for you is that walking a bit faster will actually give you an energy boost. According to Robert Kertzer, a physical fitness expert at the University of New Hampshire, brisk walking is an excellent way to promote cardiovascular fitness. It encourages the heart to work at an increased, yet safe, "exercising rate." In addition, it lowers the resting heart rate and reduces blood pressure. Because walking produces this kind of effect on the cardiovascular system, you will be getting the benefits of a thorough fitness program without risking the hazards of overdoing it.

One study reported in the journal *Medicine and Science in Sports* found that women who walked on a motor-driven treadmill for 30 minutes a day three times a week for 6 weeks showed an increase of 12 percent in maximum aerobic capacity at the end of the training period. In another study, 40- to 56-year-old sedentary men walked 40 minutes a day four times a week for 20 weeks. They showed significant improvements in resting and active pulse rates and in oxygen uptake, as well as a decrease in weight and body fat.

EASY WEIGHT LOSS THROUGH WALKING

The benefits of walking don't end at the heart. They hit you in the hips, as well. This was demonstrated quite well by a group of obese women in California who added a hearty, daily walk to their sedentary lives. The 11 women in the experiment lost an average of 22 pounds in one year. And they did it without changing their eating habits. But the researchers did note one very important thing: None of the women showed any weight loss until they got their walking routine up to 30 minutes a day—until they got their bodies working aerobically. When their weight stabilized, they simply added more walking time to their routine. And, yes, you guessed it, they started losing weight again.

The reason why walking can help you lose weight without eating less (although you can't eat more!) is a simple matter of arithmetic. The energy needs of a person sitting quietly are about 75 calories an hour. But get that person on his or her feet and on the move, and the number of calories burned can triple. Obviously, physical activity requires more energy than sitting. Activities that force you to use your legs, even only moderately, use a considerable amount of energy.

Walking definitely has its advantages over other types of exercise. For one thing, walking is about the safest exercise you can do (if you find a safe place to walk). It's also something most of us are pretty good at. You don't have to concentrate on putting one foot in front of the other, which gives you time to let your mind wander. Better yet, walk with a friend and enjoy conversation. And, if you are one of those who wants to avoid being labeled a crazy fitness freak, you can pull the wool over people's eyes by walking. It's such an innocent, normal activity.

You'll be glad to know that the list of benefits of walking is as long as your leg. In addition to burning extra calories, it improves the circulation in your legs, which helps you avoid getting varicose veins. Walking improves muscle tone in the legs, making them more shapely and healthy looking. Also, walking is a natural tranquilizer. It can reduce anxiety and tension, and even relieve depression. If you have a constipation problem, rejoice: Walking stimulates elimination and makes your digestive system healthier. Even many people with heart disease and those with arthritis or emphysema can enjoy the benefits of walking.

There are many exercises for which similar claims can be made. But none can match the ease of walking.

When it comes to your health, it's the least you can do.

Building Endurance

Walking is the easiest way to start an aerobics program. Just slip on some comfortable shoes and walk away from the house for 10 minutes, turn around and walk back. Do this 3 to 4 times during your first week, with a day off between walks. Walk as slowly as you wish. Once you've progressed to Week 4, you can start increasing your pace.

Week	Day 1 (min.)	Day 2 (min.)	Day 3 (min.)	Day 4 (min.)
1	20	20	20	20
2	20	25	20	30
3	20	30	25	35
4	25	30	30	40
5	25	35	30	45
6	30	35	35	50
7	30	40	35	55
8	35	40	40	60
9	35	45	40	70
10	40	45	45	75
11	40	50	55	80
12	50	60	50	90

Walking Warm-Ups

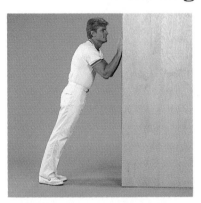

Lean. Lean on a wall without bending your knees or back. Lean forward with your elbows bent. Hold for 3 seconds and push back.

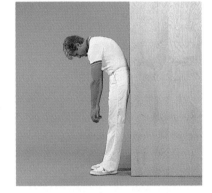

Hang. Stand with your back against a wall. Relax and let your arms hang down, pulling your shoulders and head with them.

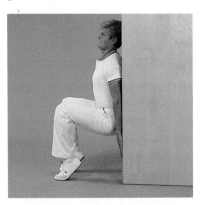

Squat. With your back against a wall, slide down until your thighs are parallel to the floor. Hold for 10 seconds.

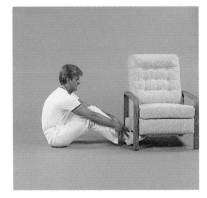

Sit-Up. Lie on your back, flex your knees and hook your feet under a chair. Slowly sit up and grab your ankles with your hands.

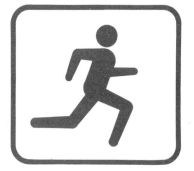

Running

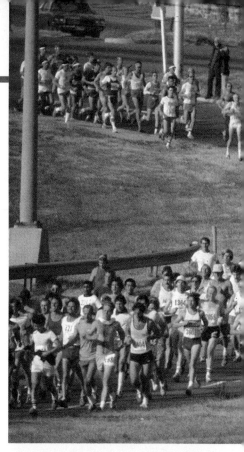

You see them everywhere these days, jogging up city streets and down country lanes—the growing number of Americans who run after health and well-being.

It's estimated that 33.3 million people in this country are avid runners. And no wonder. Running makes you look good and feel great and it gets you in tip-top shape. It's not uncommon for a good long-distance runner to have a resting pulse rate as low as 41 beats a minute!

Running also improves lung capacity and the blood transport system. It strengthens legs, muscles and bones. It reduces body fat and increases lean body tissue. And, perhaps best of all, it can help slow down the signs of aging.

It's true beyond a doubt that running is good for you. And it's true that running carries very little risk—as long as the program you follow is a sensible one. If your usual workout has been nothing more than a casual stroll in the park, you can't expect to pick yourself up and run 2 miles any more than you could walk into a gym and lift a 200-pound weight. First, you've got to get ready. If you cut corners before you start, you'll very likely pay the price in sprains and enough pain to make you wonder whether the whole business is worth it.

But such mistakes can be avoided if you keep in mind these all-important tips:

- Select good running shoes, ones that fit—and fit well. You'll feel how good (or bad) your shoes are some 5,000 times each hour you run, so don't skimp or try to make do with shoes designed for some other sport.
- Warm up before you run by easing into your pace. Strains and sprains are common injuries among runners, especially beginners. Strains and sprains are the result of stretching muscles and ligaments beyond their limit. When you warm up before running, your muscles and tendons elongate and accommo-

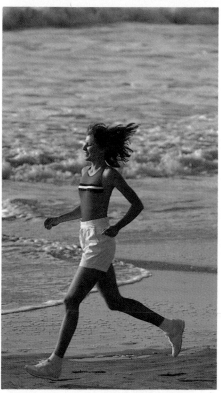

date the greater range of action that running demands.
- Follow each run with a cooling-off period: 5 or 10 minutes of casual walking and mild stretches. This will enable the blood to

(continued on page 33)

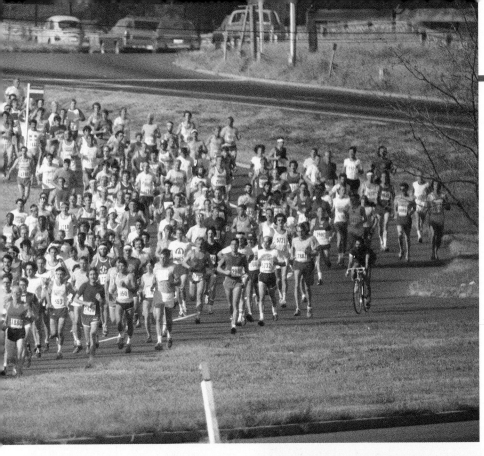

From the exhilarating start of a marathon race to the solitude of jogging beside a churning sea, running is the one sport in which the participant can make his own set of rules and always come out the winner. Runners are becoming a common sight from coast to coast.

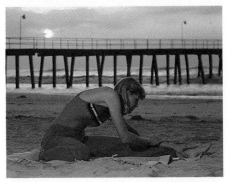

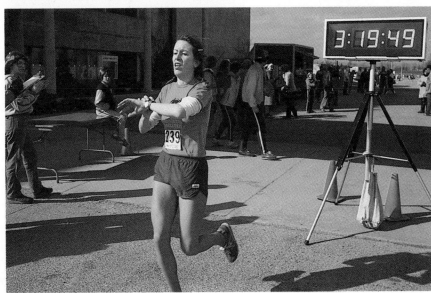

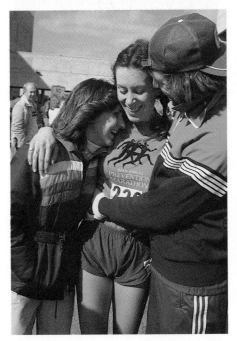

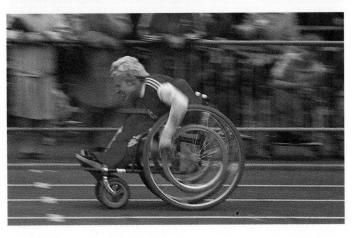

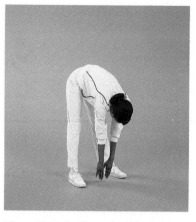

Floor Touch. Stand with your feet spread, bend at the waist and reach for the floor with your fingertips.

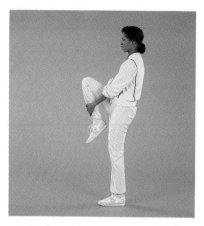

Knee Raise. Raise one leg until you can grasp your ankle. Hold for 3 seconds. Repeat with other leg.

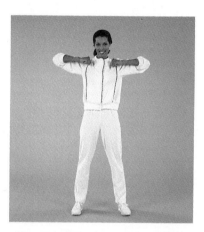

Wing Stretch. Bend your elbows and raise your arms to shoulder height. Thrust them out and back. Repeat.

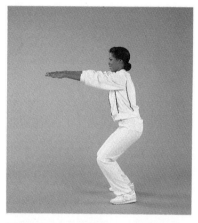

Half Squat. With your arms outstretched in front and feet slightly spread, bend your knees as if to sit, then stand up.

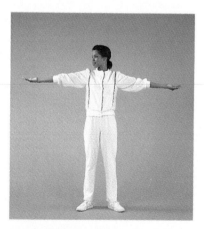

Neck Stretch. Spread your arms and move your head to look right, then left.

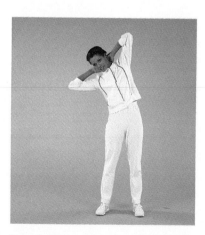

Bend. Clasp your hands behind your neck. Bend to one side and then the other.

CAUTION

Injury Is Avoidable

Many runners enjoy their workouts so much that they sometimes run too far too fast, injuring themselves in the process. But these injuries can often be avoided. Watch out for warning signs, such as pain in the knee, hip and ankle joints. If they hurt before a run, wait a few days until the pain goes away and then run more slowly than before. If the pain comes while you're running, stop and walk until the pain goes away. If it persists, walk home and put ice on the joint. If the pain doesn't subside within 48 hours, see your doctor. It may be something serious.

The same advice applies to muscle strains, except that you *can* continue to run as long as the muscle pain is only slight.

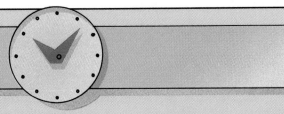

Building Endurance

The best way to start a running program is by mixing running with walking. If you're able to walk at a brisk pace for 30 minutes, you should have no trouble starting this schedule at Week 1. You'll start by walking 4 minutes, then running for 2 for a sequence of 5 times and a total of 30 minutes. This program is most successful when you do the routine 3 to 4 times a week with a day's rest between sessions. If, however, the routine seems too easy and you've completed it on 2 separate days without any trouble, you may progress to the next week's program. If you can't walk for 30 minutes, follow the walking program on page 29 before attempting the running program.

Week	Walking (min.)	Running (min.)	Number of Times	Total (min.)
1	4	2	5	30
2	3	3	5	30
3	2	4	5	30
4	2.5	5	4	30
5	3	7	3	30
6	2	8	3	30
7	2	9	3	33
8	1	9	3	30
9	2	13	2	30
10	1	14	2	30
11	1,1	20,9	1	31
12	0	30	1	30

return to your heart from your extremities without pooling and generally will ease your body's return to a resting state.

- Learn to run properly. A poor gait is the most frequent reason people have problems. Bad runners look like ducks or penguins. Don't follow their example. Keep your back straight and your head forward. If you bend forward the strain on the muscles of your back will mean a backache when you get home.

There's no question that running asks a lot from your body. But if you pursue it gradually, your body will be able to endure these stresses—and endure them well.

A sensible training program should take your age into account. If your cardiovascular system is sound and you have no joint and bone problems, there's no reason why you should stay away from the running track. Some experts advise beginners to run on alternate days, to give themselves time to rest and recover from each outing. Dr. Cooper believes that a satisfactory pace for running is 10 minutes per mile, and that a person won't benefit if he runs less than 2 miles a day four times a week. On the other hand, running more than 3 miles a day five times a week can do you harm. "I'm convinced," says Dr. Cooper, "that if a person wants to continue for the rest of his or her life to be involved in a good aerobic-type exercise program, he or she has to stay within those limits."

If you really want to get out and jog but you need a little more incentive, try this: Jogging burns about 400 calories a half hour—the amount you might find in a hot-fudge sundae. Good, hard exercise does have its sweet rewards.

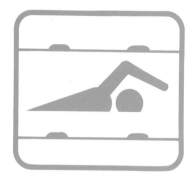

Swimming

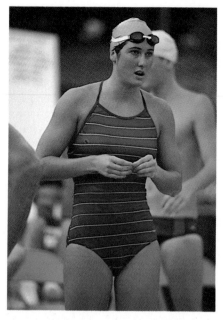

Joggers may be clogging the roadways and sidewalks, and cyclists may be whizzing by on their 10-speeds, but, very quietly, swimming also has become an enormously popular sport in this country.

The findings of a national opinion survey indicate that 13 percent of the population swims for exercise every day or almost every day. This compares with 29 percent who jog, 29 percent who do calisthenics and 28 percent who bicycle at least once a week.

Swimming ranks right up there with the tops in conditioning when it comes to improving your health. A number of swimming experiments conducted at the University of Illinois found that regular, long-distance swimming produced the same benefits as running, cycling or cross-country skiing. Another study on endurance and strength in women

When it comes to swimwear for fitness, modern design has it all over the cumbersome togs worn in 1900. The fashion of the day made even wading in the blue Mediterranean a mite difficult.

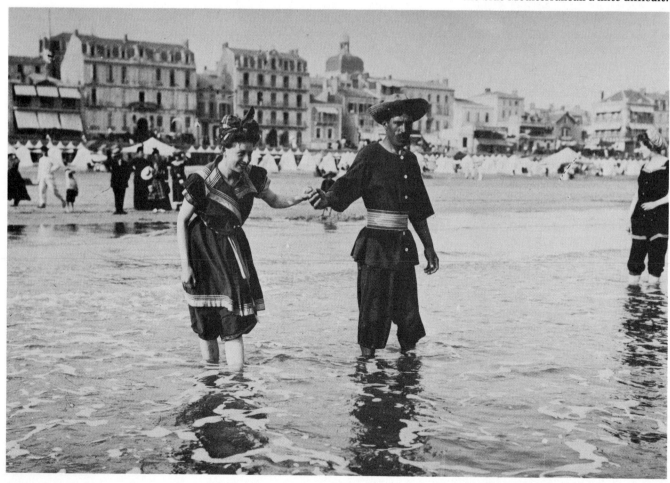

archers, dancers, fencers and other athletes found that the greatest endurance gain was made by the women swimmers. Other researchers have found that swimmers ranked higher in various fitness tests, including leg power, flexibility and cardio-respiratory endurance, than modern dancers, folk dancers and basketball players. And in the area of strength, muscle tests conducted at the University of Oregon showed that, as a matter of course, swimmers increased the strength of their calf, leg, upper back, abdominal, chest and lower back muscles.

Another great thing about swimming is that it gets you fit *fast*. Scientific studies show that you can get into good shape by swimming only twice a week for 15 minutes each time. Of course, just splashing around in the pool isn't "swimming," but you don't have to wear yourself out, either. Swim a lap (about 25 yards or meters) every minute, and you're doing as much for your heart (and much more for your arms, back and stomach) as any jogger.

And the best thing is that all these body benefits are yours without blisters, shinsplints or runner's knee. Rather than sweat you up and tire you out, swimming cools you off and relaxes you.

WATER MAKES EXERCISE EASIER

In swimming, it's not the exercise but the water that's kind to your muscles and bones. Stand in water up to your neck and you're suddenly 90 percent lighter. This means a person weighing 150 pounds weighs only 15 pounds in the water. And the body's lightness in water gives swimming a superior advantage over other sports. For one thing, this water pressure improves your circulation by 25 percent or so as soon as you step into the pool. You can't say that about your first step on the running track!

What's more, swimming isn't tough on the joints, which makes it a great exercise for people with arthritis.

"People with painful joints will usually find it possible and comfortable to move in the water," says James E. Counsilman, Ph.D., the highly regarded coach of the Indiana University swimming team. That also makes it the ideal exercise for older people. "Swimming seems to be the standard exercise for older people because many of these people, like me, can't jog because of some ache or another," he says.

And if you're overweight, the fact that swimming is non-weight-bearing means you won't have to fight gravity at every step of the way. Swimming burns 350 to 400 calories an hour—without burning you out.

AQUA AEROBICS—EXERCISE WITHOUT WEAR AND TEAR

You don't need to swim laps in an Olympic-size pool to reap all the benefits of swimming. Even a small corner of the pool will do for the great conditioner known as aqua aerobics.

Water and exercise mix well. Water helps protect you against injury while it increases the intensity of your workout.

The protection comes from the support it gives you. That's why many runners, when they're hurt and can't hit the road because of the damage caused by the road hitting them back, choose to run laps in the pool. You don't have to run too fast in the pool to get your heart rate as high as it would go during a workout on dry land. When you are immersed in water, the water acts as a giant cushion for your joints against the ravages of gravity.

Compare jumping rope on land, for instance, with jumping in a shallow pool (shallow being about waist deep). Jumping rope on dry land can be rough on your knees, ankles or hips. Every time you land, your lower body absorbs a shock equal to several times your body weight. Even the vibrations from landing can be harmful, traveling up your spine to your shoulders, arms and head.

But jump up and down in water

(continued on page 37)

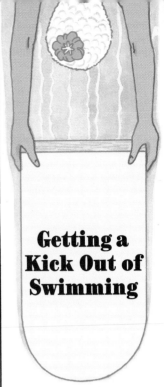

Getting a Kick Out of Swimming

A kickboard is probably the simplest and most useful exercise device for swimmers—beginners or advanced—says Jane Katz, Ed.D., author of *Swimming for Total Fitness*. It supports your upper body while allowing you to breathe normally while practicing your kicks. Simply hold the board in front of you with your fingers curled around the upper end and propel your way through the water. Or, hold the board from the bottom end so you have room to put your face in the water to practice rhythmic breathing.

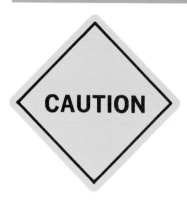

CAUTION

Before the Plunge . . .

Your eyes may wear out before your endurance does if you don't treat them with care. To prevent the inevitable sting from chlorinated water, wear a good pair of goggles. Look for a pair with padded lenses so they'll fit tightly but not squeeze so hard that they cause a headache. An adjustable nosebridge will give you an even better fit.

Also, to guard against the common nuisance known as swimmer's ear, put a few drops of rubbing alcohol in your ears after each swim. It causes water to evaporate, keeping the canals dry and clean.

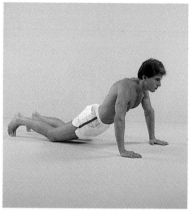

Modified Pushup. Lie on the floor with your knees touching and palms flat. Push up until your arms are fully extended.

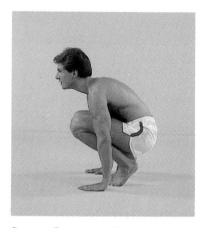

Squat. Squat until your palms touch the floor. Raise your heels.

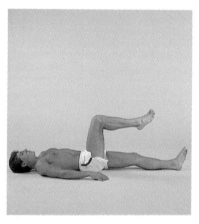

Leg Raise. Lie on your back and raise one leg at a time, flexing the knee.

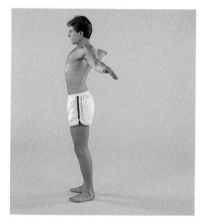

Stretcher. Stand with your arms spread like wings and gently flex them as far back as possible, then return.

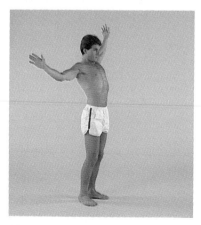

Shoulder Flex. Stand with your arms spread at the shoulder and slightly bent at the elbows. Bend toward the floor.

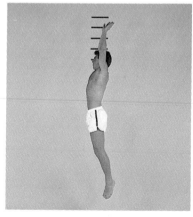

Jump. Stand with your feet together and your arms raised straight over your head. Flex your knees and jump straight up.

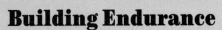

Building Endurance

The easiest way to begin a swimming program for the first time is by counting strokes. One complete stroke involves both arms, so it's best to keep count on your right armstroke. Start with 10 strokes, stop and walk 1 pool length. If you're more than halfway to the end of the pool when you complete your strokes, walk another length. If your pool has a deep end and you cannot walk the length, you'll have to get out of the pool and walk. In this case, it's best to swim in an end lane. Complete the 10 swimming strokes and walking sequence for 30 minutes. For best results perform this routine 3 to 4 times during the week with a rest day between sessions. To successfully acquire the fitness to swim for an entire 30 minutes, simply progress from Week 1 to Week 12 on the swimming chart.

Week	Swimming (no. of strokes)	Walking (pool lengths)	Duration (min.)
1	10	1	30
2	20	1	30
3	30	1	30
4	45	1	30
5	60	1	30
6	75	1	30
7	100	1	30
8	125	1	30
9	150	1	30
10	300	1	30
11	250	1	30
12	300	1	30

and most of the shock of coming down eddies out around you in the waves that slap the pool side. The same principle applies to running in the water. It's easier on your body than pounding out miles on the road. With each step, the water protects you.

Despite that, however, you'll quickly notice that it's harder to jog in water than it is on a cinder track—a lot harder. That's because water is thicker than air, and as you run, H_2O resists your motion mightily. This water resistance makes your leg muscles, heart and lungs work hard, creating an aerobic conditioning effect if you keep going long enough.

Even water games, if played at a steady clip, can be aerobic conditioners.

But can this fun help you burn calories? You bet. Researchers at the University of Georgia found that in 20 to 60 minutes of aqua aerobics, you burn a little over 6 calories a minute, making it equal to slow jogging or lap swimming.

So, it doesn't matter if you're swimming laps or doing the doggie paddle; swimming is great exercise. And you can't use the excuse that it's only useful to those who live in the Sun Belt, either. Practically every city in the country has a Y or community organization with an indoor pool.

Everyone into the pool!

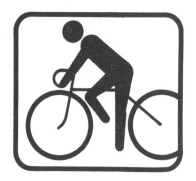

Bicycle Riding

It's faster than walking, as much exercise as jogging and it gets you there sitting down. No wonder bicycling is one of the fastest-growing sports in America!

Yes, cycling is a form of exercise you can easily learn to love. After all, what other exercise allows you to take in so much scenery, enjoy the company of family and friends and even serve as an economical way to travel? On your bike there are no lift lines, no courts to wait for. You can go almost anyplace there's a road. Unlike jogging, where your legs pound the road with every step, riding a bike is not a weight-bearing activity. The smooth, rhythmic movement is less stressful to your joints. And if you tire, you can ease up and coast, knowing you are still moving toward your destination.

Another nice thing about bicycling is that you're never too old to take it up and continue to benefit from it for the rest of your life. In fact, when it comes to physical benefits, pedal power is right up there with foot power. This was well proven at the University of California at Davis, where researchers studied the physical fitness merits of three popular forms of exercise—jogging, bicycling and tennis. Middle-aged sedentary men were assigned to participate in one of the three activities for 30 minutes a day three times a week. The experiment lasted for 20 weeks. When it came to fitness, the joggers and cyclists were equal, with both groups showing significant improvement in endurance. Not only that, but both groups also lost a substantial amount of body fat. Unfortunately, the tennis players did not fare as well. They showed only a modest increase in endurance.

GETTING STARTED

If cycling is more or less new to you, ease your way into it. Begin with half-hour rides every other day or three days a week, and give those

With all the bikes on the roads these days, it's hard not to be aware of the burgeoning interest in cycling. But the real passion for the sport is most evident among the racers and spectators who pack such places as the Lehigh County Velodrome near Allentown, Pennsylvania.

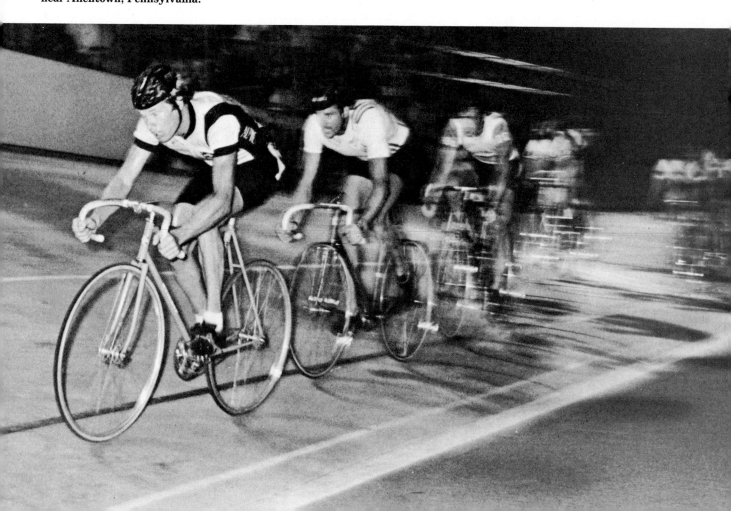

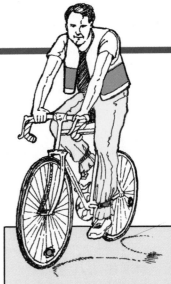

new-to-cycling muscles 48 hours to recover.

A common mistake made by beginners is that they try to kill themselves pushing the pedals at too high a gear. This is wrong. You should feel only minimal resistance, spinning the pedals lightly—about 70 revolutions or more per minute. If you pedal steadily instead of pushing hard and then coasting when you tire, you'll raise your pulse plenty high and find a pace you can enjoy. (Don't huff and puff so hard you can't carry on a conversation.) As you build endurance, you'll find you can gradually ride longer and faster. As you get stronger, you can ride every day if you want to, but alternate shorter, easier rides with longer ones so you still can rest every other day.

If you haven't ridden a bike for a while, you might want to practice a few basic skills in an empty parking lot. Learn to shift gears without wobbling and to look over your left shoulder while steering straight ahead. When you take to the roads, always ride *with* traffic; ride in the street on the right, as motor vehicles do. Be predictable: Use hand signals and ride in a straight line. Obey one-way signs, traffic lights and the like. Avoid riding so close to parked cars that a door could be flung open in your path. Finally, though you may never need it, a helmet is a wise precaution.

If you can, eliminate that gas-guzzling commute and do errands on the bike. You'll find real satisfaction in the self-sufficiency of your own muscle power and get some exercise at the same time.

Utility cycling usually means a little planning ahead. You'll need a bike bag or basket for carrying things, so you can keep your hands free for braking. A big U-shaped lock or the assurance of a safe place to leave the bike is a necessity. When shopping, you may be able to take the bike right into the store.

Commuters have the option of wearing their work clothes on the bike if the ride is short, or changing after arrival. If you choose the former, wear sensible, low-heeled shoes (not sandals) and use a pants clip to keep your trouser leg away from the greasy chain. A woman who wishes to ride in a skirt can do so with a dropped tube bike (either a "ladies" or "mixte" frame) and a seat with a short "nose" made for that purpose.

If you ride after dark, make sure you have adequate lights on the bike, reflective tape on your helmet and anything else you can come up with to make you resemble a Christmas tree on wheels. Your local bike shop should be able to help you.

BUYING A BIKE

If you are excited about going out and riding fast on your bike, the 10-speed (or more) bike, also called a derailleur bike, is for you. The dropped handlebars allow an aerodynamic position that cuts wind resistance to a minimum. But you don't have to ride bent way over all the time. The bars let you vary your hand position, so you can sit up somewhat when you want to. Theoretically, a wider range of gears is possible on a derailleur bike. Ask at the bike shop for touring gears rather than racing gears, to help you tackle the hills. Shifting is mastered easily; ask the salesperson to show you how. If you want them, fenders and a carrier can be added to this bike.

The 3-speed bike offers upright handlebars, which are built more for comfort and less for speed. Because you sit up straighter on the bike, you're much less likely to encounter a sore neck and a backache, but your position is less aerodynamic. The type of gearing on this bike means easy shifting—a bonus in heavy traffic—and easy maintenance. However, the gearing is probably less versatile than that on the racier-looking model. The 3-speed is an excellent choice for short rides and for commuting, providing your route is not too hilly. Fenders, often standard equipment, are there to cut down splash on a rainy day, and a rear carrier allows you to attach bike bags securely.

Commuting Made Easy

Buy a bike that suits your distance. Besides the traditional 3-speeds for short rides and 10-speeds for long rides, there are new fat-tire, all-terrain bikes that provide an all-purpose alternative. Put your belongings in a backpack or tie them down in a basket or rear carrier. If possible, park your bike in the office or lock it securely outside, removing all accessories. Carry a tool kit to fix flat tires and learn to use it *before* you start to ride. Wear lighter clothes than usual—your body heats up as you exercise.

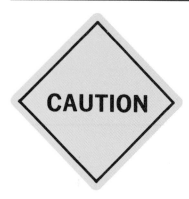

CAUTION

Get a Bicycle Built for You

An ill-fitting bike will stress your muscles and cause fatigue. The seat should be just high enough so that your knees are slightly bent when the pedal is at the bottom of the stroke. On a bike with dropped handlebars, the top of the handlebars should be about 1 inch below the saddle.

Dress for the weather, with loose upper layers and long johns under cotton shorts when it is cold. Avoid conventional trousers in almost any weather. They chafe the legs and can get caught in the chain. So can scarves and purses.

Drink plenty of fluids in hot weather—fruit juice diluted with water is good—to prevent heat exhaustion.

For a bicycle you can depend on for years, it's wisest to buy from a bike shop, not a department store. Product quality and service will be better. For a good 3-speed bicycle, expect to pay anywhere from $130 to $170. The minimum cost of a derailleur bike is in the same range—about $160. But you could pay as much as $2,500 for a superb model.

THE STATIONARY BIKE

While cycling gives you the most fun for your energy when it's done outside, it's just as effective if you do it indoors on a stationary bike.

Being able to keep a close check on the amount of work you're doing so you can accurately record your progress is one of the big advantages of stationary bicycles. Basically, they're bikes without a rear wheel, mounted on a stand, that allow you to keep track of your work effort in terms of speed, mileage and pedal resistance (which can be manually adjusted). They range in price from less than $100 to several thousand dollars (for space age affairs with digital panels).

Cycling Warm-Ups

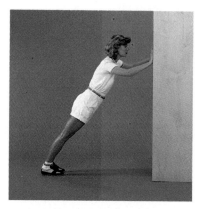

Lean. Stand with your feet about 3 feet from a wall. Lean toward the wall and push away.

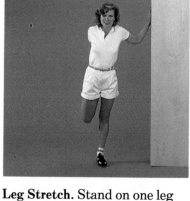

Leg Stretch. Stand on one leg and grasp your other ankle, pulling your foot up as high as possible.

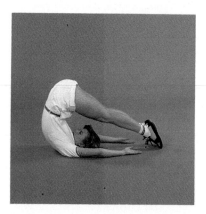

Upper Back Stretch. Lie on the floor with your hands overhead. Swing your legs over until your toes are close to or touch the floor.

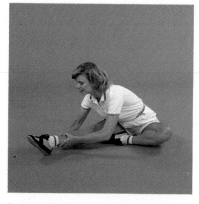

Lower Back Strengthener. Sit on the floor and rest one foot against the opposite thigh. Bend and grasp your outstretched ankle.

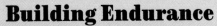

Building Endurance

The most efficient way to cycle for fitness is with a stationary bike. The reason for this is that you can pedal at a consistent cadence with a specific resistance and not worry about distractions such as dogs, intersections and hills.

To start, make sure the seat is adjusted properly and release all tension from the bike. Slowly begin to pedal and increase the cadence until you reach about 30 km/hr (18-20 mph). At this point, check your heart rate. If you're at 60 percent of your maximum heart rate continue to pedal for 20 minutes. If you're lower, increase the resistance slightly, pedal for 2 minutes and record your heart rate again. Repeat this sequence until you reach 60 percent of maximum. Follow the cycling progression from Week 1 to Week 4, completing each session 3 to 4 times a week with a rest day between workouts. Once you reach Week 4 you can increase the resistance (pedal cadence remains at 30 km/hr) so that you are at 65 percent of maximum for 1 week, then 70 percent and finally 80 percent.

If you're riding outdoors at a more leisurely pace or inside at less than 60 percent of maximum, then you should progress to Week 12.

Week	Day 1 (min.)	Day 2 (min.)	Day 3 (min.)	Day 4 (min.)
1	20	20	20	20
2	20	25	20	30
3	20	30	25	35
4	25	30	30	40
5	25	35	30	45
6	30	35	35	50
7	30	40	35	55
8	35	40	40	60
9	35	45	40	70
10	40	45	45	75
11	40	50	55	80
12	50	60	50	90

If you're in the market for a stationary bicycle, particularly if the whole family is planning to use it, you should look for a model that's not too noisy and that has a comfortable seat, a way to change the resistance, adjustable handlebars, a light but solid frame and a heavy flywheel (front wheel). The heavier the flywheel, the smoother the ride. A cautionary note: When riding a stationary bike in a closed room, your heart rate can go up very fast, so it's best to either set up a fan or open a window.

The ventilation problem is solved by one ingenious new development in fixed-bike design, in which pedaling activates a large fan and also moves the handlebars back and forth, keeping you cool and working your upper body at the same time. Also, you can exercise only the arms and upper torso by working the handlebars alone, only the arms and shoulders by working them from a standing position or only the legs and hips by pedaling alone. As a result, the machine is a sort of total body exerciser with four different exercise stations.

Probably the biggest drawback to the stationary bike is boredom, which is why you shouldn't set it up in an out-of-the-way place like a dreary basement or a musty back room. Rather, put it in a convenient place—like by a telephone. Or in the TV room. Or place a reading lamp right next to it. You can start a whole, new way of gauging your reading time. So, how many miles do you think it would take to read *War and Peace*?

Rope Skipping

If there could be a perfect exercise, what would it have to be?

It would have to be good for the heart and lungs, right? And good for muscle toning and weight loss. It would also have to be convenient to do, safe and inexpensive. And fun.

Well, hang on to your clothesline, because jumping rope, believe it or not, comes about as close as anything. That's why it's as popular with professional boxers as it is with schoolyard kids. For an activity that doesn't take you anywhere, jumping rope covers a lot of bases.

When you jump rope, you use muscles not only in your legs, but also in your arms, back and shoulders. And the more muscles any given exercise incorporates, the more blood your heart has to pump—and the more oxygen your lungs must breathe to keep these muscles moving. It's for this reason that rope skipping compares so favorably with all other aerobic activities. When rope skipping was analyzed in laboratory experiments by Dr. Ken Cooper, 10 minutes' worth proved to be the fitness equivalent of jogging 1 mile in 10 to 12 minutes; cycling 3 miles in 9 to 12 minutes; swimming 350 yards in 6 to 8½ minutes; or 20 minutes of continuous handball, basketball or squash.

That's a lot of exercise. And if you want to know more precisely the benefits that skipping rope can bestow, a study done several years ago with 10-year-old boys produced the following results: "Greater leg and knee strength, increased calf size, better jumping ability, faster running speed, greater agility and flexibility, broader shoulders and deeper chests and improved heart response." Not bad for an activity that need take you no farther than your living room.

But how good is rope skipping at burning calories? Very good. Not quite as good as running, but still right up there with most other aerobic activities. For example, 10 minutes of skipping rope (for someone weighing 150 pounds) burns approximately 100 calories. That's the equivalent of an equal amount of time spent jogging (at about a 10-minute-per-mile pace) or cycling (at about 13 miles an hour). Put another way, jumping rope burns about 10 calories a minute, for most people.

THE PORTABLE EXERCISE

If you're the type who gets bored easily by exercise, at least while skipping rope you can watch TV or listen to music. You can even keep an eye on the kids, if need be.

Perhaps the most convenient aspect of all with skipping rope, though, is its portability. If you have to do a lot of traveling, it's certainly easier to pack a jump rope than a set of barbells or a stationary bicycle. It beats running because you needn't risk getting lost (or mugged) in a strange city. Just carry your trusty little jump rope with you and you can run your own mini-marathon, if you like, without ever leaving your hotel room.

But don't let anyone convince you that jumping rope is a breeze. For one thing, it does require a certain amount of skill. And it can be hard on the ankles, knees and hip joints. So those of you with old football injuries, beware!

Also, it's important to be a little discriminating about what you choose to skip *on*. Choose something with some give to it, like a wooden floor, or a surface covered with resilient indoor-outdoor carpeting. Concrete can be quite jarring. And asphalt is only slightly softer.

And the best shoe for skipping? Any good sneaker or running shoe will do just fine.

And the rope? Well, there are ropes and there are ropes. You can spend as much as $12 or more for a super-duper leather job with wooden handles containing ball bearings for easy turning. Or you can cut yourself a length of clothesline and knot and tape the ends. What you decide to "swing" is up to you.

Happy hopping.

Building Endurance

While rope skipping is a great aerobic activity, it can be tough getting started. But by mixing rope skipping with walking you can progress to a full 30 minutes of skipping. Complete each weekly routine 3 to 4 times, with a rest day between sessions.

Week	Skipping (min.)	Walking (min.)	Number of Times	Total (min.)
1	0.5	1	20	30
2	1	1.5	12	30
3	2	1	10	30
4	4	2	5	30
5	5.5	2	4	30
6	7	3	3	30
7	8	2	3	30
8	9	1	2	30
9	13	2	2	30
10	14	1	2	30

Rope Skipping Warm-Ups

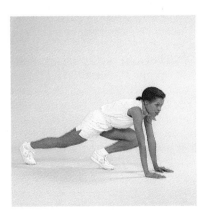

Sprinter. With palms on the floor, bend one leg forward and fully extend the other leg to the rear. Rapidly switch legs.

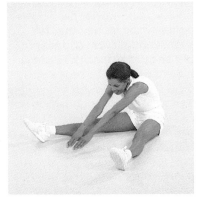

Hamstring Stretch. Sit with your legs spread, and touch the floor with your fingertips, extending them as far as possible.

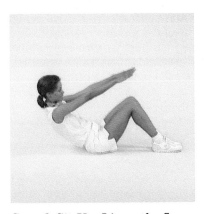

Crunch Sit-Up. Lie on the floor with knees flexed. Raise your upper body with arms extended until your lower back is off the floor.

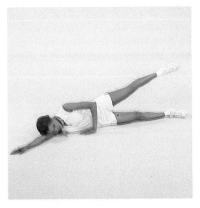

Leg Raise. Lie on your side. Raise your top leg as high as possible and lower slowly. Reverse position and repeat.

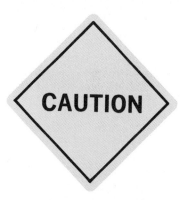

CAUTION

Jump with Joy —Not Pain

When skipping rope, wear sneakers or shoes with cushioned soles to protect your feet and absorb the shock, and don't jump on surfaces like concrete or asphalt. You can reduce the impact of a jump by jumping only high enough to clear the rope.

This exercise puts a lot of stress on your leg muscles and feet, so approach it as cautiously as if you were out for a long jog.

Aerobic Dancing

Remember the last time you enjoyed kicking up your heels on the dance floor, your mind lost in the rhythm of the music? The time flew by. You could have danced all night.

Did that seem like exercise?

Of course not. And that's why aerobic dancing has become so popular. Dancing is fun, and the music helps you forget that what you're really doing is exercising. The aerobic part simply means that while you're dancing continuously, you're also raising your heart rate.

Aerobic dancing consists of a mixture of rhythmic running, hopping, skipping, jumping, sliding, stretching and swinging, as well as a wide variety of dance steps. The dances are usually choreographed to fit a particular piece of music that ranges from ballroom dances and jazz to polkas and ballet. The routines are supposed to be easy for the beginner and challenging for the experienced exerciser at the same time. Fortunately, dancing skill and technique are not critical. Even those who can't dance can catch on to aerobics.

A study at North Texas State University used a group of 31 women to determine whether aerobic dancing is vigorous enough to raise the pulse rate significantly. The 12-week program consisted of 30 to 40 minutes daily of continuous movement—either reviewing dances, learning new ones or walking and jogging between dances. The researchers found that the resting heart rates of the dancers were significantly lower at the end of the experiment.

In another study, the participants performed six routines of 3½ minutes each at low, moderate and high speeds on different days. The dance sessions were separated by short recovery periods of walking, jogging or dancing practice. The results showed that the energy expenditure for the moderate sessions was comparable to ice skating at 9 miles an hour, walking at 3½ miles an hour, or bicycling at 10 miles an hour.

THE AT-HOME ROUTINE

Dance-exercise classes are available in most cities. But there's no reason why you can't "get into gear" at home. A workout should include: a warm-up, starting out slowly and gradually picking up the pace; vigorous movements, which could be running in place, jumping up and down or dancing; shaping and toning exercises to firm the muscles; and a final series of easy stretches and breathing exercises that help you relax your muscles and keep them from stiffening.

But, before you can begin your workout, you need to find music with a consistent beat. Put on slow tunes for the warm-up and cool-down and upbeat, jazzy music for the fast moves.

Then find a pace that's comfortable for you. If you pick the right music, it will pace you. You won't have to concentrate. You don't want to go too easy, but you don't want to get out of breath, either. Find a pace that allows you to breathe easily.

And then don't forget to breathe. Lots of people hold their breath when they exert themselves. You should concentrate on breathing deeply and fully. "I tell people to breathe in like they're sniffing a rose and out like they're blowing out a candle," one instructor advises.

Stay tuned to your own body so you'll know when to take a break. But don't forget to stretch before you stop completely. Otherwise, you might end up with sore muscles. Once you get the swing of it, you can adapt any exercise to music. Do calisthenics, or make up movements as you go along. There are dance instruction books and records available to help you add variety to an at-home workout.

Remember to keep moving for at least 15 to 20 minutes. If at first you find that too difficult, don't be discouraged. Within a week or two you'll notice an improvement.

Building Endurance

Like jogging, brisk walking, swimming and cycling, aerobic dancing is an exercise intended to condition your heart. But unlike these other exercises, aerobic dancing isn't the type of conditioning program you can ease into easily.

Most people do aerobic dancing with a group headed by a very energetic and athletic instructor. And even though there are warm-up and cool-down periods, any normal beginner will find it a bit hard to keep up. About the best thing we can recommend is to find a program *for beginners*. This should help you get used to aerobics at a slower pace. Also, there are beginners' records that you can buy to follow at home.

If you're totally out of shape, it might be wise to start getting in shape by following one of the other programs suggested in this chapter, like walking or running, and save your yen for aerobic dancing until you know you can keep your pace up for a half hour.

Aerobics Warm-Ups

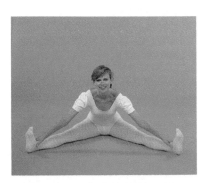

Hamstring Stretch. Sit on the floor with your legs spread. Bend and grasp your ankles.

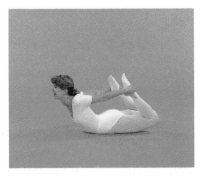

Turtle. Lie face down on the floor. Raise your chest and grasp your ankles, pulling your feet toward your buttocks.

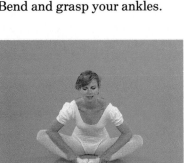

Hip Stretch. Sit with the soles of your feet together and close to your body. Use your elbows to press your knees toward the floor.

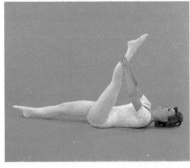

Hip Flex. Lie on your back and raise one leg until you can grasp your ankle. Switch legs and repeat.

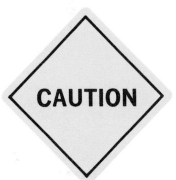

CAUTION

Swing Slowly to the Pace

There is dancing, then there is *aerobic* dancing. And Kenneth Cooper, M.D., sees a problem with the style of dance designed to get you into cardiovascular shape. That problem: Trying to keep pace with the instructor. "Not going through a proper beginners' program can be dangerous," cautions Dr. Cooper. Start at half-pace, if that's what is comfortable for you. Don't strain to try to keep up with a group that was active for a long while before you stepped in.

Rowing

When you think of rowing, what image immediately comes to mind? Slaves in galleys propelling ancient vessels of war? Viking explorers? English gentlemen competing at Henley-on-Thames on lovely summer afternoons? Ivy League college crew teams?

Rowing is all that and more.

Rowing is, in fact, one of the most versatile and accessible aerobic sports. We're talking about rowing as a sport—for competition or exercise— not meandering around in a rowboat. It's being practiced by men and women of all ages in ever-increasing numbers, according to the United States Rowing Association (U.S.R.A.). Its pluses are numerous.

- It's a great aerobic exercise for people with orthopedic problems because it doesn't place a great deal of stress on joints.
- Rowing exercises most of the large muscle groups of the body.
- You can do it in your home or office with the help of a rowing machine, which simulates the water's resistance with tension devices.

To move through the water, rowers use their upper bodies and arms to take long, powerful strokes with oars. Their feet are tied into shoes attached to the boat's bottom. They intensify their strokes by using their legs to move back and forth on sliding seats that roll on a track about 2½ feet long inside the boat.

Rowing builds strength and endurance. "It ranks among the most physiologically demanding of any aerobic sports, with cross-country skiing being its only parallel," says Frederick C. Hagerman, Ph.D., an exercise physiologist at Ohio University. Why? "Because of its high endurance factor and the stress placed on muscles by repetitions," he says.

GETTING STARTED

If you decide to take the plunge, your best bet would be to join a rowing club and take lessons there, using the boats they have available.

The U.S.R.A. publishes a listing of its many member rowing associations, if you want to find out where the nearest club is. In most clubs, members' ages range from 12 to 70 or older. They row in everything from sleek racing boats to recreational boats. The U.S.R.A. is located at #4 Boathouse Row, Philadelphia, Pennsylvania 19130.

You can also join the U.S.R.A. without joining a local club. The membership entitles you to enter any of the U.S.R.A.-registered regattas, which are boat races held on various rivers around the country. The association will help you out with instructional films, regatta schedules and equipment listings. Competition among master rowers is one of the association's fastest-growing areas. But recreational rowing, for the sheer exercise of it, also is expanding rapidly.

If you choose not to go the club route, you'll have to think about buying your own boat. Although boats were once phenomenally expensive, the newer fiberglass ones cost as little as $1,000 to $1,200 for a single (one-man) scull. (Sculls are boats propelled by two oars per man, as opposed to sweeps, which are boats with one oar per man.)

Since most people don't have ready access to open water, the most widely used equipment for rowing is found in the gym and the home. Rowing machines are designed to allow you to imitate the arm, leg, back and upper body action of actual rowing. And you get the same aerobic benefits available from rowing on the water.

The better machines have a moving seat that slides when you pull and push the oars and a means of adjusting the resistance so that you can increase the intensity of the exercise. Some have an ergometer for measuring speed and the distance you've rowed.

No matter where you choose to do your rowing, you can count on a pretty good caloric output. Vigorous rowing can use up about 600 calories an hour and an easy row about half of that.

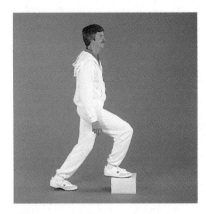

Building Endurance

If you're taking up rowing for the first time, start with a rowing machine. Begin by mixing rowing (12 to 20 strokes per minute) with walking. From the second week through Week 12, mix brisk rowing (20 strokes per minute) with recovery rowing of 12 strokes per minute. Complete each routine 3 to 4 times weekly with a rest day between workouts.

Week	Rowing (min.)	Recovery (min.)	Rowing (min.)	Recovery (min.)	Number of Times	Total (min.)
1	3	2	0	0	6	30
2	3	2	0	0	6	30
3	4	1	0	0	6	30
4	4	1	3	2	3	30
5	4	1	0	0	6	30
6	4	1	5	1	3	30
7	9	1	0	0	3	30
8	13	2	0	0	2	30
9	14	1	0	0	2	30
10	20	1	9	0	1	30
11	25	1	4	0	1	30
12	30	0	0	0	1	30

Rowing Warm-Ups

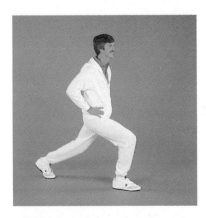

Stride. Step forward as far as possible, keeping the back straight. Return to the starting position and switch feet.

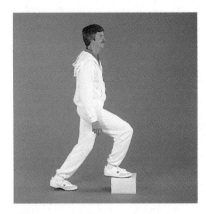

Step-Up. Step up and down on a block of wood or a step. Switch legs each time.

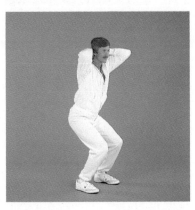

Squat. Place your hands behind your head and squat as if you're going to sit in a chair.

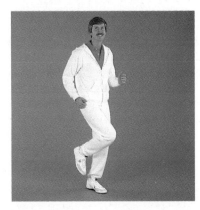

Jog. Jog in place with arms up for 100 steps. One step is complete when left foot hits the floor.

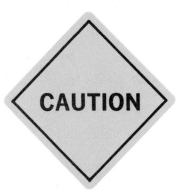

CAUTION

Tips for the Crew

Blisters. They're a minor but persistent problem for rowers. Says Kathryn Reith of the United States Rowing Association, "they're something every beginner must endure," and gloves won't help much. But, says Ms. Reith, "you'll start to build up calluses after a while."

Warning: This is not a sport for poor swimmers. Although boats can capsize easily, life preservers aren't worn because they prevent freedom of movement.

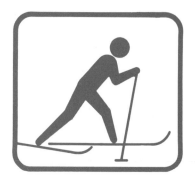

Cross-Country Skiing

Do you want to enjoy winter the way you did as a kid? Then slip on a pair of cross-country skis. Cross-country skiing is a Scandinavian sport that's gaining a reputation in this country as a fun way to get through the snow.

If you hate downhill because of its chill, you'll appreciate the constant warmth you'll feel when you ski cross country. Cross-country skiers break into a comfortable sweat even in freezing weather. There are no lift lines to wait in, no cold rides to the top of the mountain. And there's no tedious learning process. Cross-country skiing, also called Nordic skiing or ski touring, is becoming more popular because *anyone* can do it.

Of all forms of exercise, cross-country skiing might be the most complete. Because you use both your arms and your legs, and because you're usually carrying heavy clothes and equipment, you get roughly twice as tough a workout as you would by jogging or walking at the same speed.

Technically, cross-country skiing is known to require more oxygen than almost all other kinds of exercise. It's comfortable, though, because it demands a lot of small exertions instead of a few big ones.

It's also an excellent aerobic exercise, according to Edward G. Hixson, M.D., chief physician to the U.S. Nordic Ski Team that participates in the Olympics. "First, it's very good for the heart and lungs. It's more strenuous than running, but you don't have to go real fast.

"Second, it's a relatively pain-free exercise. There are no aches and pains, there's no pounding on the pavement. Your heel doesn't take any shock, and there's not as much stress on the knees as in running."

Skiing is also a great way to burn calories. A person at rest burns about 75 calories per hour. But a good skier burns up to 1,000 calories an hour. The average skier would fall somewhere in the middle of this range, depending on how fast he skis.

IF YOU CAN WALK, YOU CAN SKI

Unlike a downhill skier, you don't need to learn fancy techniques if you want to get to your destination in one piece. The general principle employed to move forward is *walking*. It's that simple. But skiing is more fun than walking because you can glide between steps. When you really become

Skiing Warm-Ups

This series of exercises is designed to warm up the body for the unique movements skiing requires. From left, raise your arms straight out to your sides and press them to the rear; with feet 45 degrees to the side, twist from side to side; with your feet together, push your buttocks back and lean forward, keeping your arms outstretched behind you; flex your knees and jump straight up; flex your knees again and twist your upper body from side to side; with feet together and knees bent, jump and turn 90 degrees while in the air.

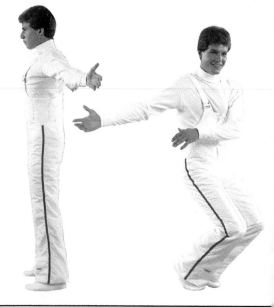

Building Endurance

A cross-country skiing program is much like a running program. In place of walking and running, you'll start out by combining beginners' learning techniques with skiing. Once you're skiing for the full 30 minutes, it's time for a harder workout. Move back to the first step and alternate slow and brisk skiing.

Step	Learning/ Slow Skiing (min.)	Skiing/ Brisk Skiing (min.)	Number of Times	Total (min.)
1	4	2	5	30
2	3	3	5	30
3	2	4	5	30
4	2.5	5	4	30
5	3	7	3	30
6	2	8	3	30
7	2	9	3	30
8	1	9	3	30
9	2	13	2	30
10	1	14	2	30

adept, you'll develop graceful, flowing movements that can move you along quite fast—even up hills.

You don't need much to become a Nordic skier. For the first time on snow, you can rent skis, boots and poles for less than $10 a day. That way you can find out if you like it. Once you're hooked, you can be outfitted for less than $150. An equivalent package for downhill skiing, by comparison, costs roughly $400 to $450. Nordic skiers also avoid the expensive lift tickets that downhillers must buy.

Also, you don't need a lot of special clothing to go ski touring. The important thing is to wear several thin layers of clothes rather than one bulky jacket or sweater.

So scout out a trail—in your backyard or in the city park, on a riding trail, a hiking or biking path or an unplowed road. More and more resorts are developing cross-country trails near their downhill areas. The trails are usually marked for novice through expert, depending on the number of hills. Another good thing about these areas: They have "groomed" tracks—tracks pressed into the snow to make gliding easier.

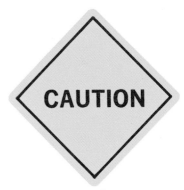

Think Comfort Head to Toe

Dressing for the trail calls for lots of layers so you can easily shed a tog or two as you begin to work up a sweat.

Also, properly fitting boots and bindings are essential. Have only a qualified person fit your equipment. Ill-chosen footwear can lead to serious injury in a fall.

And, watch those thumbs! The most common injury in this sport is "skier's thumb," which comes from trapping the thumb between the strap and the grip of the pole during a tumble.

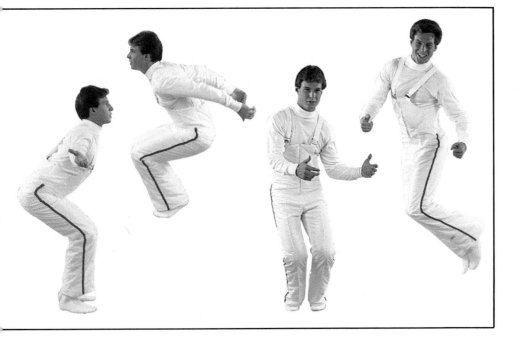

49

4

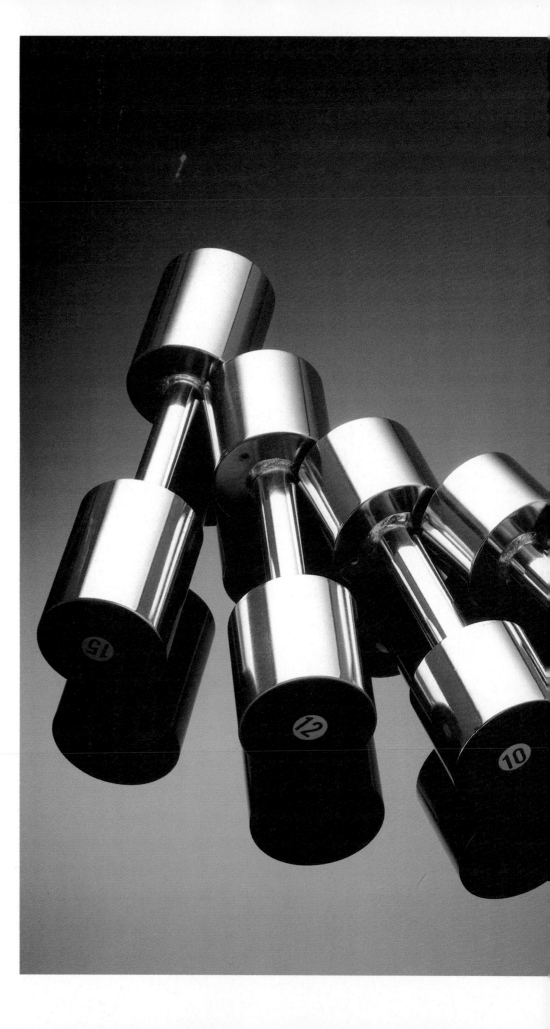

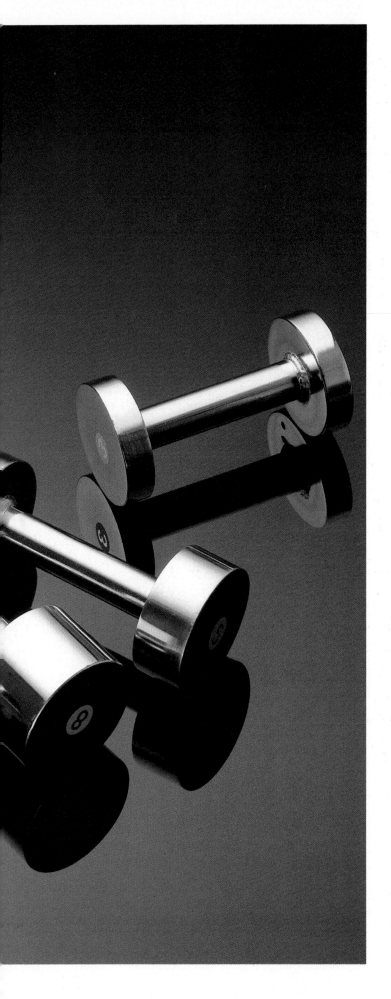

Building the Body Beautiful

Weight lifting's not your style? Think again. It can mean a more shapely and energetic you!

Muscles are beautiful, says the new age of fitness.

That is not to say that the beautifully fit person must have arms like tree trunks. But shouldn't we at least have arms that can chop one down should the occasion arise? Shouldn't we have legs with something between skin and bone? Shouldn't we be able to carry our own luggage from the nether regions of the parking lot (Q-5!) to the check-in counter?

Strength—*pure physical strength*—is often required in order to do what our spirit wills us to do—whether it's jetting away to Antigua or walking through 9 inches of snow on a moonlit night. That's the real beauty of strength. It empowers you—a personal bill of might.

It doesn't look too bad, either. Six months on a strength-training regimen may not send a man to the loincloth department of his favorite haberdashery, but it may well send him from the full-cut shirt counter to the tapered. Where it will send the newly firmed and trimmed woman is limited only by her imagination.

If you're wondering just what strength training entails—which we hope you are—here's a quick definition. Strength training is an exercise program that involves working the muscles against gradually increasing degrees of resistance. It differs from exercises such as jogging and racquetball—which obviously also give your muscles a workout—by employing the "overload principle." That is, a conscious effort is made at several points in the workout to challenge the muscles with more resistance than they can comfortably handle for more than a few repetitions of the exercise. Muscles respond to the regular employment of overload challenges by steadily increasing in strength and sometimes in size as well.

The only women who want to look like female body builders are female body builders. The rest of the female population would rather have muscles that are firm and shapely—but small. Weight lifting, however, can get you to your goal. Don't worry about ending up with muscular biceps and triceps "by accident." The exercise that gave this woman her competitive shape requires an unusual amount of dedication and time.

In jogging or racquetball, by contrast, the degree of resistance is almost unchanged from week to week. In such activities, strength usually increases rapidly after the sport is begun, but tends to plateau very quickly.

What are the benefits of strength training to those of us who have no intention of ramming a quarter ton over our heads in a weight-lifting contest, or flexing "pecs" that look like living falsies in a Mr. Universe contest? There are lots of benefits, it turns out. Benefits that can help women and men—old, young and in between.

STRENGTH ENHANCES SELF-RELIANCE

You may enjoy excellent cardio-respiratory fitness and a high degree of flexibility, but neither of those qualities is going to make it possible for you to change a tire, bring in an armful of firewood, bust the sod to plant a garden, tote your own luggage or carry a slide projector from one end of an office building to the other.

Greater strength is especially important to today's working woman. All those men who smiled and insisted on opening the heavy door for you may have been closing the door of opportunity right in your face. Many jobs in public safety, for instance, require that women pass the same strength and agility tests that men take. Business-women who must travel are at the mercy of cab drivers and porters unless they can carry a suitcase, a briefcase and a shoulder bag all at the same time for at least 15 minutes. And the self-defense courses women take can be pretty meaningless unless there's enough oomph behind that kick to get the point across.

The weaker you are now, the more you stand to gain from strength training.

STRENGTH TRAINING SLOWS AGING

One of the inevitable consequences of aging is a gradual loss of muscle mass. The result is that by the time you are over 40 or 50, your strength may be drastically less than it was at 20. By 65, a woman who has followed a sedentary lifestyle may have no more strength than a child. Fatigue comes easily, everyday tasks become monumental chores. Posture poops out, and you begin to think of yourself as old even though your mind may be as young as ever.

Strength training is just the ticket to combat this slide into premature senescence. While it's probably not possible for a person of 60 to maintain the same muscular strength he or she enjoyed at 20, it is definitely possible for a fit 60-year-old to enjoy the strength of the average 45-year-old or for a 45-year-old to have the power of a 25-year-old.

If you have never followed a strength-building program before, you can actually throw the deterioration of your muscles into reverse gear by starting one now. You'll be building muscle instead of losing it. As each day passes and you continue your workouts, your muscles will in effect become younger and younger. Eventually you'll reach a limit to this rejuvenating effect, but by that time, you'll be well ahead of the game.

Loss of muscle mass isn't the only loss we suffer with age. Both men and women also lose bone mass as they gain years. The process begins earlier in women—often by age 25—and progresses more rapidly, too. But both sexes suffer from the problem—osteoporosis—and its consequences can be fearful: chronic back pain, vertebral collapse and broken hips. Once again, strength training can come to the rescue. Contrary to what you might think, working against resistance builds not only muscle, but bone, too. It's believed that muscular contraction around bone somehow stimulates it to conserve its structural minerals. Tennis players, for instance, have been found to have not only larger muscles but also thicker bones in the arm with which they hold the racquet. A training regimen that includes every muscle group in the body can therefore be expected to have profoundly beneficial effects on the strength of the skeletal system.

GREATER STRENGTH MEANS GREATER ENDURANCE

The increased mass and strength of a trained muscle group does more than give you the ability to unleash a sudden burst of power. Most people used to think of strength training in those restricted terms, but researchers have shown that besides being strong, trained muscles can keep putting out work over a period of time with much more efficiency and less fatigue. That's why you'll find a wide range of athletes from long-distance runners to boxers training with weights these days. The benefit is there even if the athlete never uses the full strength of his or her muscles in one all-out burst of power.

In a sense, it's a *reserve* of strength that's helping them. It's impossible for any machine—including the human machine—to put out power to the absolute max over an extended period of time without suffering premature wear and tear on its parts. Strength training gives you a new, higher max. Now translate that principle into your golf game or lap swimming or country rambling and what you get is less fatigue, better performance and the next day, less muscle soreness.

The reserve tank of power for your tennis or golf game doesn't disappear when you leave the court or fairways. It accompanies you to work, follows you home and gets into bed with you. A hundred different everyday tasks and activities suddenly seem slightly less difficult. But even that slight difference can change a feeling of "what next?" into "how about it?"

MUSCLES HELP YOU LOSE WEIGHT

Have you ever marveled at the amount of food that some teenagers

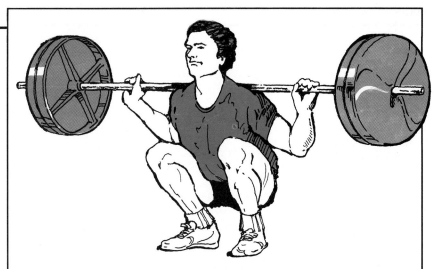

Male Strong Points

While records in almost all sports are starting to equalize as women realize their fitness potential, there's one area where differences are almost sure to remain—weight lifting. It's a physiological fact that, in general, men have greater upper body strength than women. Take a look at the gap between men's and women's records for the snatch, a maneuver in which a weight is thrust overhead; for the clean and jerk, a similar maneuver in which the weight is held momentarily at shoulder height before being thrust overhead; and for total poundage.

Men's Records
Weight Classes (as of 7/1/83)

Event	123 lbs. (56 kg.)		132 lbs. (60 kg.)		148 lbs. (67.5 kg.)	
	Weight (lbs.)	Name	Weight (lbs.)	Name	Weight (lbs.)	Name
Snatch	239.8	Albert Hood	254.2	Phil Sanderson	293.9	Cal Schake
Clean & Jerk	296.1	Charles Vinci	337.0	Issac Berger	361.3	Michael Jacques
Total	530.4	Charles Vinci	574.6	Issac Berger	640.9	Nicholas Vernucci

Women's Records
Weight Classes (as of 8/21/83)

Event	123 lbs. (56 kg.)		132 lbs. (60 kg.)		148 lbs. (67.5 kg.)	
	Weight (lbs.)	Name	Weight (lbs.)	Name	Weight (lbs.)	Name
Snatch	144.8	Mary Beth Cervenak	133.7	Diane Redgate	171.3	Judy Glenney
Clean & Jerk	194.5	Mary Beth Cervenak	193.4	Jane Camp	215.5	Judy Glenney
Total	337.0	Mary Beth Cervenak	320.4	Jane Camp	381.2	Judy Glenney

can put away without showing any evidence of their gluttony? That phenomenon is often passed off as "fast metabolism," a mysterious (and wonderful) condition that just as mysteriously (and unwonderfully) becomes "slow metabolism" in the portly adult. Well, there may be *some* inevitability behind that sad change, but a lot of it can be attributed to fading muscles, not fading years.

Muscle tissue, you see, has a faster metabolism rate than fatty tissue, *even when at rest*. That means more calories are burned away, 24 hours a day.

What typically occurs after a period of strength training is that— assuming your weight remains constant— your body gains a higher percentage of muscle and a lower percentage of fat. If you *lose* weight over a period of training, the difference is even more pronounced, because nearly all the weight you lose on a strength program is fat, not muscle. In any event, the net result is that more of the calories you eat are being diverted to maintaining your greater proportion of muscle tissue, with fewer calories left over to cause mischief. That a 40-year-old can enjoy the metabolism of a 15-year-old is probably too much to hope for. But

we do have every reason to expect that regular strength training can be of great help in stopping the weight-creep so many of us experience as adults.

MUSCLES PROTECT AGAINST INJURIES

It may never have occurred to you that muscles are built-in safety pads, but orthopedic surgeons know it all too well. A person with very little muscle mass between skin and bone to absorb the shock of a fall or other potentially serious injury is that much more likely to suffer a broken or severely bruised bone. A strong arm, quickly extended, may prevent the impact from occurring in the first place, or at least reduce its severity. These two protective functions are important at any age, but they become increasingly valuable protection to anyone who wants to pursue an active lifestyle as long as possible.

Strength is beautiful. Not just in the metaphorical sense of making you more energetic and self-reliant, but in the most literal sense as well. We aren't talking about 19-inch biceps or a 52-inch chest. We are talking about arms and legs that

The Fitness Machines

Be it a Universal or a Nautilus, you're bound to get a good workout. The Universal in the photo at right is a compact, self-contained army of weights and pulleys that is still standard equipment in many gyms. The Nautilus system,

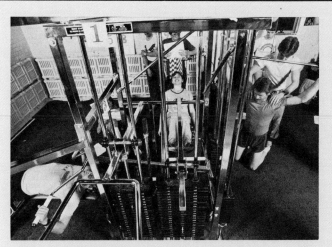

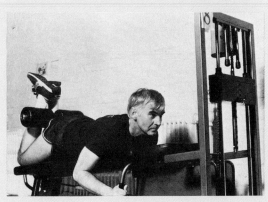

popular in many fitness clubs, has a bevy of machines, like the one shown at left, designed to work on one isolated muscle group at a time. Both work by lengthening and shortening the muscles.

don't look like they've had their vital substance sucked out. We are talking about shoulders that don't slump, posture that doesn't sag. We're talking about strong abdominal muscles that hold your stomach and intestines behind your belt without any artificial restraint.

No matter where you look, good muscles look good.

STRENGTH TRAINING CAN BE AEROBIC

Traditional weight-lifting routines or other forms of resistance training are not aerobic in nature because the relatively short bursts of work are separated by rest periods of equal or even longer length. But there's no reason why you can't design a strength regimen that improves your cardiorespiratory fitness at the very same time it's developing your muscles.

The answer is a program usually called circuit training. The idea is simple. Instead of working out against such high resistance that you require a long period of recuperation between exercise sets, simply use less resistance but move briskly from one exercise to the next.

In circuit training, the idea is to get your heart pumping but not pounding, and keep it in that healthy aerobic zone for the whole workout. The rest period between exercise sets should be no longer than about 15 seconds. The first set might be an exercise that works the chest muscles. Fifteen seconds later, you might do a set of leg exercises. Then something that works the back. Biceps. Shoulders. Abdominal muscles. Side muscles. Forearms. Neck. All of which might take you less than 10 minutes. But don't stop there. Go through the whole routine one more time. If you're huffing and puffing too much, take longer breaks. That's not cheating at all, because the idea, as we said, is to keep the heart pumping at a vigorous but safe speed. If you need a longer rest, it's because your heart is probably beating too fast. If you get through two whole series of circuit training exercises, you're doing very well. When you can do three, you're F-I-T!

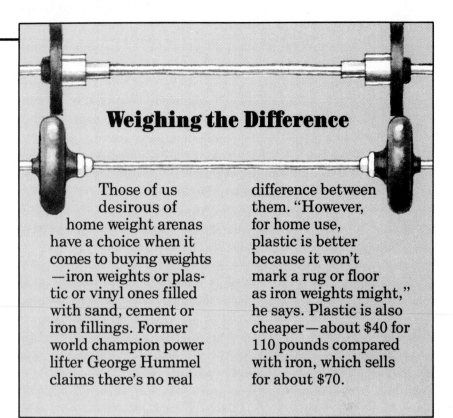

Weighing the Difference

Those of us desirous of home weight arenas have a choice when it comes to buying weights —iron weights or plastic or vinyl ones filled with sand, cement or iron fillings. Former world champion power lifter George Hummel claims there's no real difference between them. "However, for home use, plastic is better because it won't mark a rug or floor as iron weights might," he says. Plastic is also cheaper—about $40 for 110 pounds compared with iron, which sells for about $70.

HOW TO BEGIN POWERING UP

Let's take a look now at what resistance training looks and feels like in actual practice, and how you can actually enjoy all those benefits we've talked about.

Until recently, most resistance training was carried out either in gyms devoted exclusively to weight training or in the weight rooms of Y's, which were usually not particularly attractive or comfortable. Today, however, innumerable clubs catering mostly to racquet sports have installed resistance training rooms, complete with elaborate equipment often costing tens of thousands of dollars, wall-to-wall carpeting, mirrored walls and piped-in music. Unfortunately, the one thing such rooms *don't* have is a full-time instructor or coach. Typically, there is someone to show you how to use each apparatus, and perhaps to hand you a printed sheet or two with some instructions, but after that, you're pretty much on your own.

If you feel insecure about resistance training, you might want to investigate a specialized body-building studio, where you can get all the assistance you need, including gratuitous motivation in the form of

One of the greatest aids to any exercise program is visible progress, and the best way to determine if you're making progress is to keep a record of your measurements. When you see those numbers change on your chart you'll find yourself motivated to keep at it even though at times all your effort seems to go unrewarded. Here is an actual chart of a woman's progress over a 9-month stretch. Experts suggest making entries once a month or once every 2 weeks.

men and women who have made pumping iron a way of life. On the other hand, you may find the presence of such devotees to be more intimidating than motivating — especially when the grunting and groaning begins. In which case, it's back to the weight room at the racquetball club or spa.

Another alternative is to buy your own equipment and work out at home. Many people do this quite successfully, and, especially for the first six months to a year of training, there is no reason why the results achieved should be any less impressive than those obtained at a regular gym. The major drawbacks are that many of us don't really have a

suitable space to work out at home, and that in order to buy equipment necessary to exercise all parts of your body with reasonable convenience and safety, you may have to make an initial investment of anywhere from about $200 to $500.

Our advice is to begin your resistance training at a multipurpose gym. If you decide after a few weeks that weight training isn't for you, you can always play racquetball or swim, so your investment won't be wasted. More important, perhaps, is that working out in a bright, clean, fully equipped gym is usually a lot more fun than clanking around in your basement. Fitness without fun is a recipe that often falls flat.

Charting Your Exercise Progress

Date	Weight (lbs.)	Chest, Relaxed (in.)	Waist (in.)	Hips (in.)	Right Thigh (in.)	Right Calf (in.)	Right Upper Arm (in.)	Neck (in.)
1/4	176	43	35	43¼	26¼	15¼	13¾	13½
2/1	174½	42¼	34¾	43	25	15¼	13¾	13½
3/8	166	41	32¾	41½	24½	14½	13½	13½
3/22	163½	39½	31¾	40½	24¼	14½	13	13½
4/26	160	39½	31½	40	24¼	14½	12¾	13¼
5/17	153½	39½	31½	39½	24¼	14½	12¾	13¼
6/14	151	39½	31	39	24¼	14½	12½	13
7/26	150	39½	28¾	39	23	14¼	12	13
8/23	149	39	29	38½	23	14¼	12	13
9/20	147	39	28¾	38¼	22¾	14¼	12	12¾

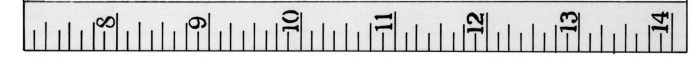

Warming Up

I t's important that you approach any exercise routine with a series of warm-up exercises. By starting your activities slowly you accomplish 3 things. You warm the muscles by increasing circulation to the muscle tissue, preparing the body for vigorous exercise. You prevent injuries and soreness. And you improve your overall performance. Make 5 minutes of stretching a routine part of your program.

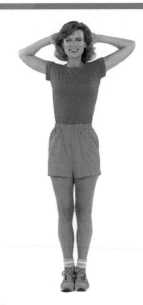

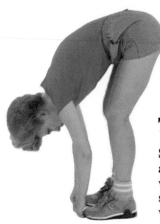

Toe Touch

Stand with your feet together and your arms at your sides. Bend slowly at the waist, bending the knees a little at the same time, until you can grab your toes with your fingers. Stand up and repeat.

Twist

Stand with your feet together, your back straight, and your head up. Place your hands behind your head and twist your upper body left and then right, moving your elbows as far as you can to either side.

Sprinter

From a pushup position, bring one leg forward until it is under your chest and your foot is flat on the floor. Quickly change the position of your legs in a continuous movement.

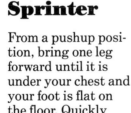

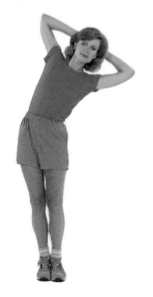

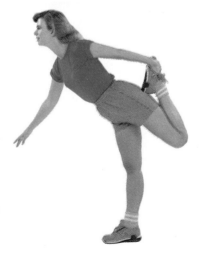

Quadriceps Stretch

Stand with your feet together and raise one leg to the rear until you can grab your ankle or your sneaker with your hand. Pull your foot toward your buttocks as far as possible without straining. Relax and repeat with the other leg. You can use a wall or a chair for balance if necessary.

Bend

Stand with your feet together and your back straight. Put your hands behind your head and bend as far as you can to the right and then to the left.

Barbells and Dumbbells

The barbell and dumbbell exercises described here are designed to build muscle, improve muscular strength and endurance and firm the entire body. This combination of exercises works every major muscle.

Squat

Bend at the waist and grasp the bar in an overhand grip (palms down). Flexing the knees, stand up, curl the bar to your chest, press it overhead and lower it to your shoulders. With feet spread comfortably and toes pointed outward for balance, squat slowly until your thighs are parallel to the floor. Return to the standing position. Try to keep your back and head straight throughout, and be sure to keep your feet flat on the floor.

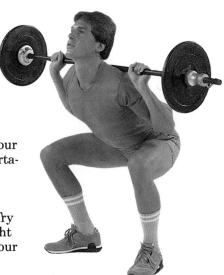

Toe Raise

Lift the bar to your shoulders as in the squat exercise, keeping your back straight and your head up. Raise your heels off the floor as far as possible. Return to the starting position.

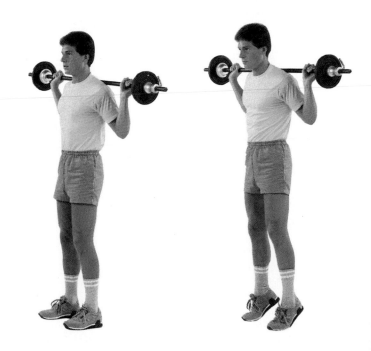

Curl

Stand with your back straight, your head up and your feet slightly spread. Grasp the bar in an underhand grip (palms up) with arms fully extended. Then slowly curl the bar up to your chest. Hold for a count of 2 and lower it slowly to the starting position. Be careful to lower the bar slowly rather than letting it drop from its own weight. Keep the bar under control at all times.

Dead Lift

Bend at the knees and grasp the bar in an overhand grip. Stand up, bringing the bar with you and letting it hang with arms fully extended. Make sure your back is straight and your head up when you are in the standing position.

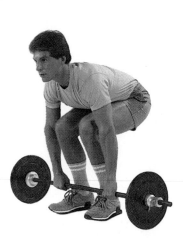

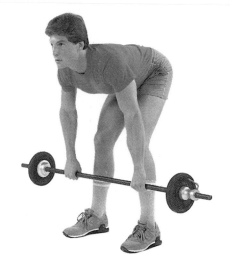

Upright Row

Stand with your back straight and your head up. Hold the bar in an overhand grip with arms fully extended. Keep your hands about 6 inches apart. Slowly raise the bar along the front of your body until your hands are under your chin. Lower it slowly to the starting position and repeat.

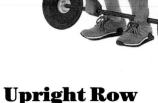

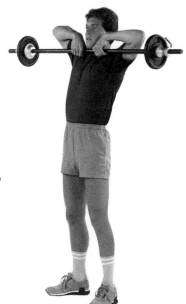

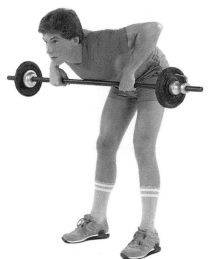

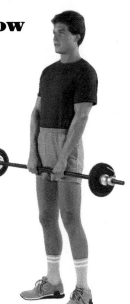

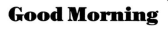

Bent Row

Bend over at the waist, keeping your back as flat as possible and your head up. Grasp the bar in a widely spaced overhand grip and raise it slowly to your chest. Lower it slowly to the floor and repeat. Bend your knees if necessary.

Good Morning

Stand straight with the bar on your shoulders and your feet comfortably spread. Then bend over at the waist until your chest is parallel to the floor. Keep your back as flat as possible throughout this exercise. *Caution:* Do not attempt this exercise if you have back problems.

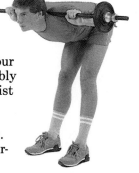

Bench Press

Lie on your back on a bench or the floor with your back flat against the surface and the bar over your chest. Slowly press the bar straight up until your arms are fully extended, then lower it slowly to the starting position.

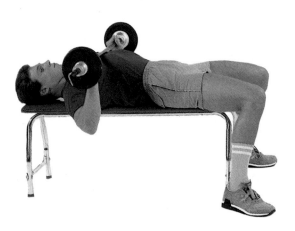

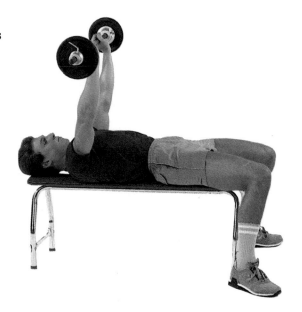

Triceps Extension

Stand erect with the bar pressed straight overhead. Your hands should be about 8 inches apart. Then lower the bar slowly behind your head by bending your elbows. Slowly raise the bar to the starting position and repeat.

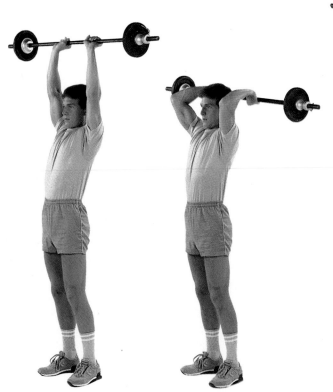

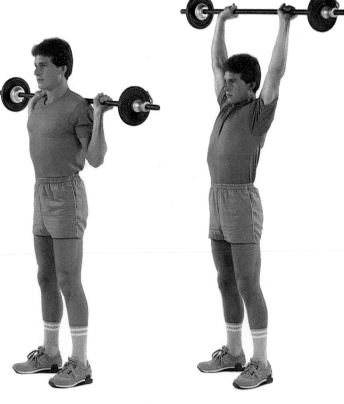

Press behind the Neck

Stand erect with the bar resting on your shoulders. Press the bar directly up over your head and lower it slowly to the starting position.

Dumbbell Press

Stand with your feet comfortably spread and a dumbbell in each hand at shoulder level. Alternately press one dumbbell and then the other straight up, with your arm fully extended.

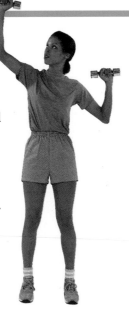

Dumbbell Swing

Stand with your legs spread and hold the dumbbell directly over your head with both hands. Then swing the dumbbell in a wide arc down in front of you and between your legs as far as you can without straining. You'll have to bend your knees to do this properly. Reverse the process and swing the dumbbell back up to the starting position.

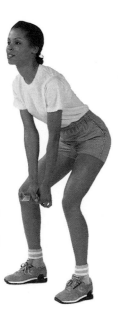

Shoulder Extension

Lie flat on a bench or the floor with the dumbbell held in both hands behind your head. Keeping your arms straight, bring the dumbbell to a position over your chest. Return to the starting position.

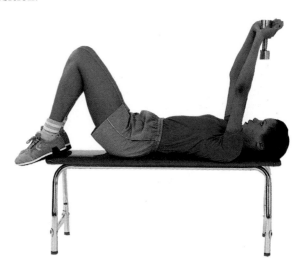

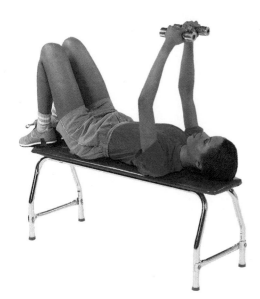

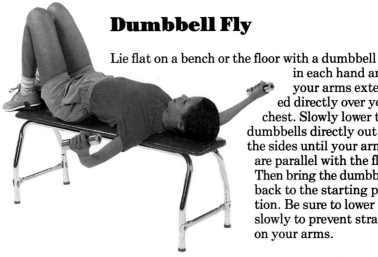

Dumbbell Fly

Lie flat on a bench or the floor with a dumbbell in each hand and your arms extended directly over your chest. Slowly lower the dumbbells directly out to the sides until your arms are parallel with the floor. Then bring the dumbbells back to the starting position. Be sure to lower slowly to prevent strain on your arms.

Nautilus and Universal Gyms

Ten years ago, the average weight-training club had all the charm of a steel mill. The floor was littered with barbells, many of them so loaded with weight that just removing enough pounds to make them liftable for the new user was a workout in itself. There was also a din of clanking as exercisers banged dumbbells together over their heads or chests, and reverberating *Booms*! as power lifters dropped hundreds of pounds of metal on ancient wooden platforms.

But such scenes are rapidly disappearing, as many gyms convert to either the Universal or Nautilus system of resistance training.

DIFFERENT APPROACHES TO THE SAME END

The Universal Gym is by far the simpler of the two, even though it looks like a Rube Goldberg creation.

When you work out with the Universal, you push or pull against bars connected to levers or pulleys, which in turn are attached to stacked weights. To change the resistance, all you need to do is remove a steel pin from one hole and insert it in another. And there is no chance at all of dropping 90 pounds on your kneecap, because the weights are confined in the "body" of the mechanism.

The Nautilus approach is radically different—and looks it. A Nautilus gym may have from 6 or 8 to as many as 20 specialized machines, each designed to work out specific sets of muscles. Looking like a cross between ultramodern furniture and medical devices, a roomful of Nautilus-type equipment can easily cost as much as two or three Cadillacs. But its advocates say it's worth it.

The biomechanical philosophy of Nautilus equipment is that while barbells and the like are simply heavy, clumsy weights, Nautilus

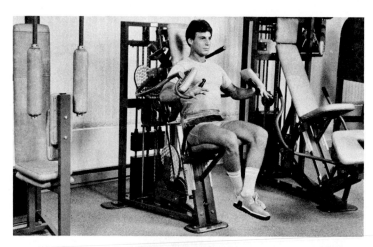

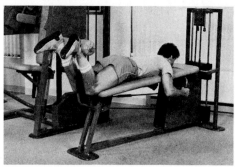

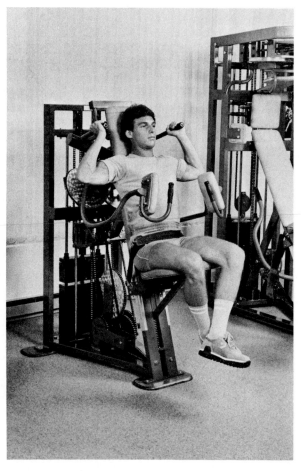

equipment is specifically designed to accommodate human musculature through a wide range of motion. What does that mean translated into sweat?

THE BENEFIT IS BALANCE

Let's say that you want to give the pectoral muscles of your upper chest a good workout using dumbbells. A popular exercise for doing this consists of lying flat on a padded bench, with a dumbbell in each hand. Just getting yourself into this position can be awkward and stressful. Then, with the arms slightly bent, the weights are lowered to the sides, until they are just a few inches below the level of the bench. At that point, the stress on your muscles (and joints) is relatively great, and the effort of moving them up again is very great. But once your arms have reached about a 45-degree angle, the effort diminishes rapidly, reaching the null point as the two weights meet over your chest. The resistance diminishes so rapidly, in fact, that the dumbbells often smash together. The result is an unbalanced exercise.

To perform essentially the same exercise with Nautilus equipment, you don't have to load any dumbbells or get them in position for lying down on a bench. All you do is stand with your back against a machine, press the inner side of your forearms against two large pads on opposite sides of your chest, and then move your arms inward until the two pads touch each other. That sounds very undramatic (and quiet, too!). But what's happening behind you is pretty exciting. There, a system of cams and chains is performing automatic adjustments to provide a constant level of resistance to your chest muscles throughout the entire range of the exercise, from beginning to end. The result is more balanced development of strength and muscle mass. And, as with the Universal Gym, resistance levels can be changed in seconds.

In many ways then—including muscle development, safety and convenience—Nautilus seems to be a superior method of resistance training. However, unless you have a very large spare room and a very large bank account, you will have to go to a club to use Nautilus equipment. Barbells and dumbbells (or free weights, as they're called) can be purchased for home use for a fraction of the price of Nautilus equipment, and stashed in a closet when they're not being used. So in some ways, they are actually *more* convenient.

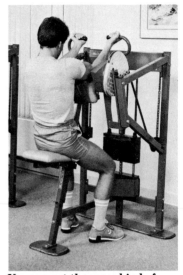

You can get the same kind of workout on a series of Nautilus machines as you can with barbells and dumbbells, but the machines are better in at least 2 ways—they are designed to make sure that you perform each exercise through a full range of motion, and they make it possible to do each exercise in the proper form and in exactly the same way each time. Each machine isolates and exercises one muscle group at a time. There are more than 20 machines designed for individual workouts. So while you can get a complete workout on a Nautilus, you're going to have to do it at a facility that has a full line of machines.

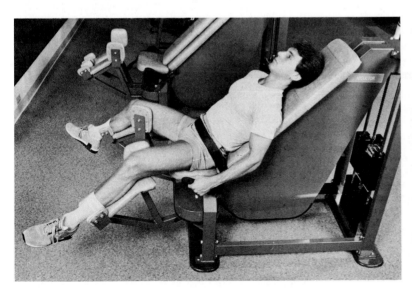

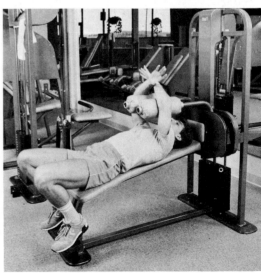

Body-Shaping Techniques

Spot *reducing* is a popular notion that unfortunately does not work, no matter how hard *you* do. Spot *building*, on the other hand, definitely *does* work.

Just how far you can take the concept of self-sculpting your body is another question. There is little question that muscle enhancement occurs most rapidly in males between the ages of about 15 and 25, thanks to the peak levels of male hormones during those years. In older men, muscle enlargement proceeds somewhat more slowly. By age 50, a man who has not previously done resistance training has no chance of ever looking like Hercules, although with any luck, he might wind up looking like Hercules' father.

What about women? It used to be said that women, regardless of age, could not develop large, rippling muscles because the right hormones weren't there. Now that many women have taken up body building as a hobby, that statement can no longer be made so glibly. Women *can* have large, even dramatic-looking muscles, although for sheer massiveness they aren't in the same league as men's muscles.

Body sculpting, or body building, as it is more commonly known, involves different exercises—in fact, a whole different philosophy—than exercising for pure brute strength. Basically, the person seeking great strength as his or her major goal will work out with relatively heavy weights (once properly warmed up, of course) and perform only a few repetitions at a time, typically three to six. And, again generally speaking, the exercises performed will concentrate on the muscles of the trunk, back, chest and hips, with a secondary emphasis on the major muscle groups of the arms and legs.

Body builders take a different route. They usually use lighter weights but do more repetitions, typically between 8 and 15, but sometimes going as high as 25. And they generally perform a much greater variety of exercises to make sure that every muscle in the body is thoroughly exercised.

Most body builders have such elaborate routines that they cannot complete an entire workout in one day. One day they may do ten different exercises for the upper body, repeating each exercise or "set" from three to six times. On the next day, they may work the muscles of the legs, abdomen or back. That approach not only enables the body builder to work every muscle, but permits an important day of recuperation for each muscle, too. (Recuperation days are important to every resistance trainer, because stressful exercise actually produces minor damage to muscles even as it encourages their growth.)

The high number of repetitions performed by body builders is what leads to the striking increase in size and visibility, or what's called definition. After performing several sets of exercises, the body builder's muscles become engorged with blood and feel hot and stiff—"pumped," as they say in gyms. But still more exercise sets for the same muscles may follow, even though the muscles now have become so fatigued that they can handle only little more than half the weight they were working out with 20 minutes before. Yet, this is exactly the part of the workout that body builders feel does them the most good and produces the most dramatic results.

For most of us, though, three or perhaps four sets of any given exercise are all we need to stimulate impressive muscle growth.

Exercising while on a space mission isn't easy. But along with their tricky maneuvers outside the space vehicle, our astronauts do manage to put in the all-important daily 30-minute workout on a specially designed treadmill. Astronaut Bill Thornton, M.D. (who manned shuttle flight 8), designed the treadmill with shoulder cords and wall handles to keep the star travelers down-to-earth about exercise. Muscle and bone loss is a problem in the weightlessness of outer space, which is why exercise is so important.

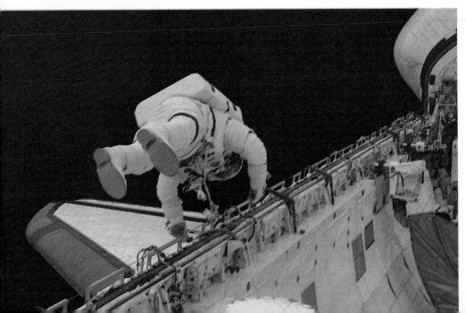

Isometrics

There's hardly a person who has never heard of Charles Atlas, the legend who raked in a pretty penny a generation ago through the mail-order sale of his easy body-building program. The program, in fact, was somewhat easy. It's called isometrics, which is nothing more than resistance against resistance.

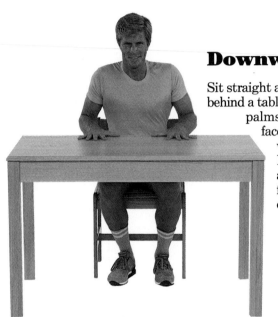

Downward Press

Sit straight and comfortably behind a table and place your palms flat on the surface about shoulder width apart. Press hard against the table for 6 to 8 seconds. Relax.

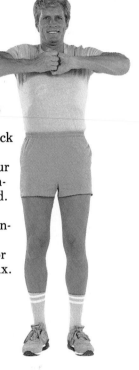

Front Grip

Stand with your back straight and your arms in front of your chest, with your fingers tightly clasped. Pull strongly outward without loosening your grip. Continue the tension for 6 to 8 seconds. Relax.

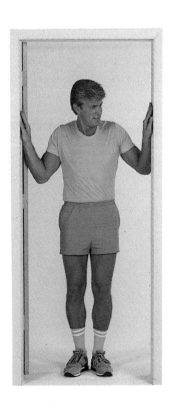

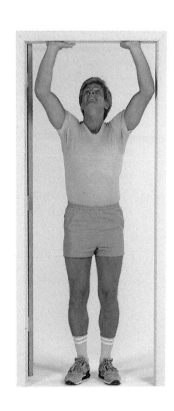

Side Press

Stand in a doorway with your hands pressed against the sides at about shoulder height. Press outward and hold for 6 to 8 seconds. Relax.

Upward Press

Stand in a doorway with your arms extended overhead and your palms flat against the top of the door frame. Press upward and hold for 6 to 8 seconds. Relax.

Gain without Strain

So there you are, standing in front of a pulley device called a lat machine, or a nest of gears, chains and handles called a Nautilus machine, or maybe just a rack of old-fashioned dumbbells done up in stainless steel so they won't look too out of place with all the other space age decor. *Now what?*

The diversity of resistance training equipment is so great today that it's beyond the scope of this book to tell you how to use each piece. That's a job for a knowledgeable instructor, or at least an experienced user. But what we *can* tell you is how to avoid cutting short your adventure in Hercules Land by making one or more common mistakes.

TAKE THE 'LIGHT' APPROACH

First, realize that weights are much heavier than they look. Or even *sound.* The reason for the deceptive heaviness of weights—which is seldom appreciated—is that in our everyday activities, we usually handle heavy jobs with lots of body English, so that the muscular strain is spread out over a whole network of muscles and bones. In the gym, though, *all* the strain tends to be absorbed by a very localized muscle group and its associated ligaments and tendons. Joints, particularly, are vulnerable to such sharply focused strain. The trick is to begin with levels of resistance *far below* what you might imagine a person in your physical condition ought to be able to handle.

There is another reason for beginning with very light resistance. Although you may proceed through your first workout without any real feeling of strain, perhaps even surprising yourself at your level of ability, you may well find that the next day, or even two days after your workout, your muscles have become extremely sore. This delayed reaction to exercise stress may well bring your fitness program to a complete halt before it's even gotten under way.

When doing any resistance exercise that involves the legs or lower back, our advice is to be not just cautious, but *super cautious.* The chance of eventually developing a severe muscle strain in the lower back is great.

Here are some more tips to keep you out of trouble, all from experienced lifters and body builders.

- When lifting any weight from the floor, always keep your back absolutely straight. And keep your neck in a straight line with your back. Don't look down at the weight; look at the wall in front of you. And put your feet as close to the weight as you can comfortably manage before lifting it. This basic technique is of crucial importance for preventing back strain.

- If you are using free weights— that is, barbells or dumbbells loaded with individual plates— make extra sure that the inside and outside collars holding the plates in place are securely locked. Even if a loose plate doesn't fall on your foot, the sudden shift of resistance and your efforts to compensate for it can bring on instant muscle strain.

- *Never* hold your breath while performing exercises against resistance. Many people do this instinctively, but it's dangerous, especially for older people. To get out of the bad habit, begin the new habit of audibly breathing in during the easy part of the exercise, then breathing out loudly during the more difficult part, such as when pressing weight over your head.

- Avoid performing any exercise in such a manner that it causes great stress in the shoulder and armpit area. Such strain occurs when, for instance, you are working with a weight-loaded bar that you pull down behind your neck from overhead. The most dangerous part of this exercise is when your arms are fully extended. In that position, a great part of the weight is no longer being handled by your muscles, but by the connective tissue around your armpits. The

(continued on page 68)

The Body Builder

Biceps

The easiest way to bigger biceps is with the barbell curl. This exercise is performed by raising a barbell from the extended-arm position to the chest. The curl should be done slowly, especially through the downward movement.

Chest

There are several good exercises to develop the chest (pectoral) muscles. The bench press is one of the most popular. To bench press, lie flat on a bench and grasp the bar overhand with your hands a little more than shoulder width apart. Lift the bar straight above your chest until elbows lock. Pause, then lower the bar to your chest.

Waist

There are really only a few exercises that directly benefit the waistline— sit-ups, leg raises, twists and side bends. For sit-ups, lie on your back with your knees flexed and then sit up. For leg raises, lie on your back, using your arms for support. With knees slightly bent, lift both legs at the same time to a position just short of perpendicular. For twists, stand with your legs apart and extend your arms to the sides. Twist the torso as far as possible from side to side. For side bends, put your hands behind your head and bend to each side. Keep your feet apart, your legs straight and don't lean forward or backward.

Thigh

To develop the thigh muscles (quadriceps) use a combination of running or biking plus squats and leg presses. Squats are performed by bracing a barbell on your shoulders and slowly squatting as if sitting in a chair. Leg presses can be done with a machine by lying on your back and pressing a weighted platform up and down with your feet.

Shoulder

The shoulder muscles can be worked with a combination of upright and bent rows and bench presses. Use an overhand grip for all exercises. The upright row is performed by raising a bar from an extended position to the chin, and the bent row by raising a bar from the floor to the chest while bending at the waist.

Triceps

The triceps muscles on the backs of the upper arms should be exercised to balance the development of the biceps. One exercise that will help do the job is the triceps extension, performed by lowering a weight behind the head as far as you can from an arms-extended position overhead, then raising it again.

Back

Exercises for the back include squats, dead lifts, and bent-arm pullovers. For dead lifts, bend at the waist and knees, pick the bar up overhand from the floor and return to the standing position with the bar at arms' length. Pause and slowly lower the bar back to the floor. For the pullovers, lie flat on an exercise bench with your head hanging off the edge. Grasp the barbell in a narrow overhand grip while it is resting on your chest. Move the barbell comfortably behind your head, holding your elbows close together.

Calf

The calves also benefit from running or biking, but the best calf exercise is the toe raise. Hold dumbbells at your sides or place a barbell on your shoulders. Lock your knees and raise up as high as you can on your toes. Hold that position for 2 seconds and then lower yourself. The calves can take a lot of work, so don't hesitate to exercise them.

strength of this connective tissue does not increase at anywhere near the speed of your muscles. Thus, after a few weeks, you may find yourself using levels of resistance that your back muscles can pull down, but that your connective tissue can't bear when your arms are fully extended. It's a lot like putting yourself on a medieval torture rack, and an injury can be very painful and take a long time to heal.

To prevent an injury while still getting benefits from this exercise—an excellent one, by the way, for developing the muscles that give you a V-shaped back—follow these two tips. First, start light—use a comfortable amount of weight and do extra repetitions. When you feel ready, move to a heavier weight. Second, when doing this or any other exercise that you sense is pulling at your joints, never work with a level of resistance that forces you to put out maximum effort.

- While it's fun and helpful to your motivation to keep track of your progress, don't fall into the habit of trying to break your personal records at every workout. Although you may find yourself doing just this—successfully— for a few weeks, you must realize that unrelenting competition— even if only with yourself—is bound to result in injury.

- Unless you are extraordinarily fit, it's best to avoid lifting weights immediately after jogging. Your circulation will be severely taxed, and you will probably find yourself deeply fatigued after your workout.

- The final tip is not for the protection of your body but of your bank account. Beware of paying a full year's dues to any body-building club in advance, particularly if the club is new. That's especially true if the club is exclusively for strength training. Multipurpose athletic clubs seem to have a better record of longevity. Also, don't pay a year's dues before the place even opens on the promise of a big discount. The club may never open at all!

We're not trying to discourage you with all these words of precaution. The point is only this: The slower you go on a day-to-day basis, the faster progress you'll make month by month.

Trying to rush things will only bring on injuries that can make progress discouragingly slow. Resistance training is an exercise designed for tortoises, not hares.

Taking It Easy

Weight lifting can cause trouble with muscle strains, a strained back or overly sore muscles if you don't learn how to control the weight. Trying to jerk the weight into position, tugging it off the floor and letting it fall out of control after a movement is completed can have serious consequences. The idea is to use smooth motions, taking only about 1 second to lift the weight and about 2 seconds to put it down.

Cooling Down

Cooling down after exercise is just as important as warming up before a workout. For one thing, your pulse rate has been elevated during exercise and it needs time to adjust to the lower demand. Cool-down exercises also help decrease muscle soreness and increase muscle flexibility. Begin these exercises with 2 to 3 minutes of walking.

Toe Touch

Sit upright on the floor with your legs extended. Begin with your hands on your hips. Tighten your stomach muscles, bend at the waist and reach for your toes with your fingertips. Hold for 10 seconds and repeat.

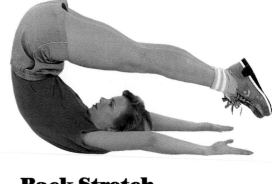

Back Stretch

Lie on the floor with your arms extended behind your head. Swing your legs over your head until your toes are a few inches from the floor.

Groin Stretch

Sit on the floor with the soles of your feet together and your arms resting on your lower legs with your elbows near your knees. Hold your feet together with your hands if necessary. Bend forward at the waist and slowly press your knees toward the floor with your elbows. Take it very easy and don't strain. Slowly move back to the starting position and repeat.

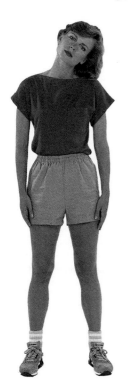

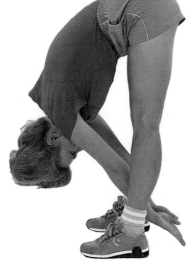

Neck Stretch

Stand with your back straight, your feet about shoulder width apart and your arms hanging loosely at your sides. Move your head slowly to one side and hold for 10 seconds, then move it to the other side and hold. Repeat, trying to bend a little farther each time.

Swing

Stand upright with your arms extended over your head and your legs spread. Begin to move your hands in an arc as you bend at the waist. Swing your hands between your legs as far as you can without bouncing. Touch the floor behind your heels if possible. Retrace the arc to the starting position.

Gimmicks and Gadgets

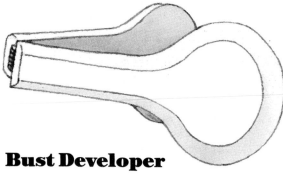

There are countless manufacturers out there who want to slim your bulging belly by thinning out your wallet. From the novice to the pro, those wanting to lift weights and work out have almost as many gadgets to choose from as ice cream lovers have flavors. But when it comes to those shiny metal and leather gizmos, not all that sparkles is good. Here's a guide to some great and not-so-great items.

Isokinetic Aid

This exercise device is designed to improve muscle tone, strength and cardiovascular efficiency. Its most famous users have been the Skylab astronauts. Like astronauts, those who have a limited amount of space and time may find the isokinetic exercise very useful. A traveling businessperson, for instance, could use this portable device in a hotel room—provided he or she is instructed about how to use it beforehand.

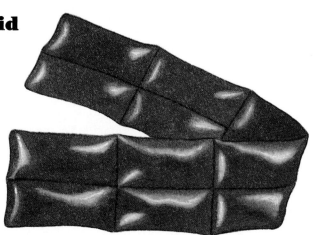

Weighted Belt

Putting on a 10-pound belt to jog or exercise is a minimally effective way to work the body harder. The same effect can be obtained by running up an incline, and you won't need to spend a dime. The principle's the same as working the body against gravity. Our advice: Don't buy it.

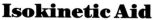

Bust Developer

About the only thing a bust developer builds up is the hopes of the person buying it. Unfortunately, the tape measure will never match its expectation. A women's sports research expert states unequivocally that bust developer exercises do not increase mammary tissue. Likewise, a study at the University of Arizona of 34 women who underwent a 21-day development program found absolutely no benefits.

Head Strap

Made of canvas, the head strap is a small harness and chain designed to hold barbell plates. It also can be attached to a pulley. Its purpose is to strengthen and develop the neck. To get the maximum benefits, be sure to get proper instructions before you attach the barbells or pulley and charge ahead. It's not a device recommended for the novice.

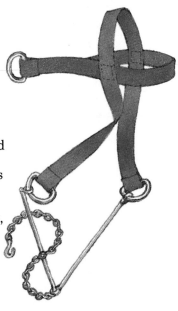

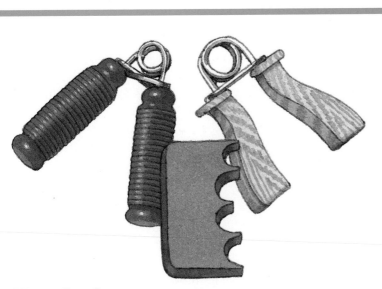

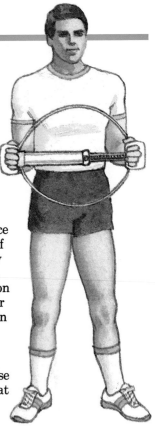

Bullworker

If you want to tone your muscles by flexing and pulling, this device can do the job—if it's used properly and consistently. But don't count on it for getting your heart and lungs in shape. This type of exercise won't get your heart pumping and pulse going the way that jogging, cycling and walking do.

Handgrips

People who work out sometimes concentrate on a few muscle areas and ignore many others. Often, they end up looking trim and toned in places like the stomach, and out of kilter somewhere else. The purpose of Handgrips is to develop the forearm and strengthen the wrist and finger grip. Making such muscles stronger can probably help your racquetball or tennis game, since strong muscles translate into more endurance. Even hauling luggage or getting grocery bags out of the trunk may not seem like such an overwhelming task.

Exercise Wheel

Exercise wheels are advertised as an easy way to trim the midriff. While they do put stress on the stomach muscles when rolled back and forth on the floor, they hardly get at the "gut" of the problem. In other words, they do nothing to rid the body of fat. Tightening stomach muscles is one way to fight the battle of the bulge, but ultimately, only exercise and diet work directly on body fat. This device may have appeal as a quick, fun way to slim down, but it may be just a way of putting off the real work of losing weight.

5

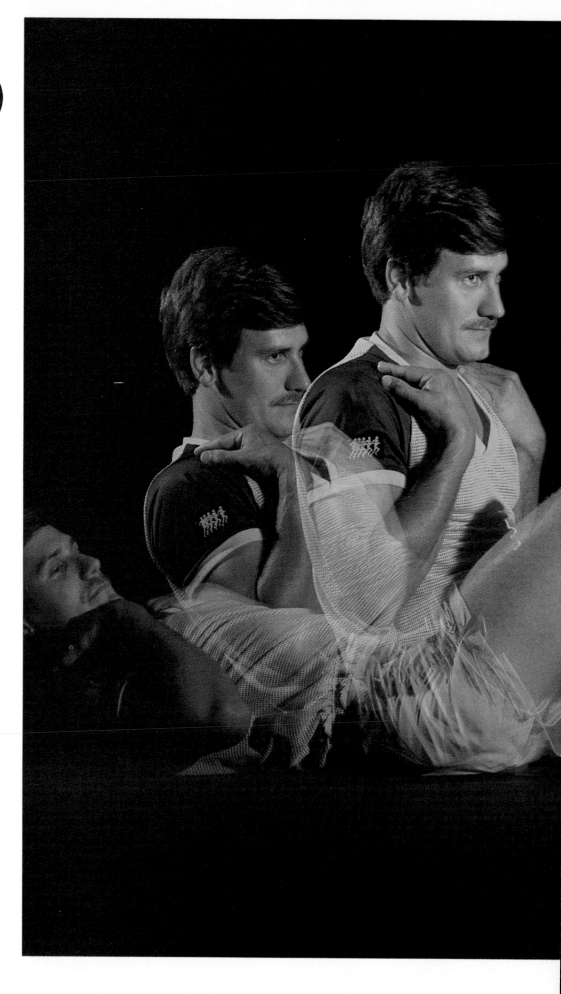

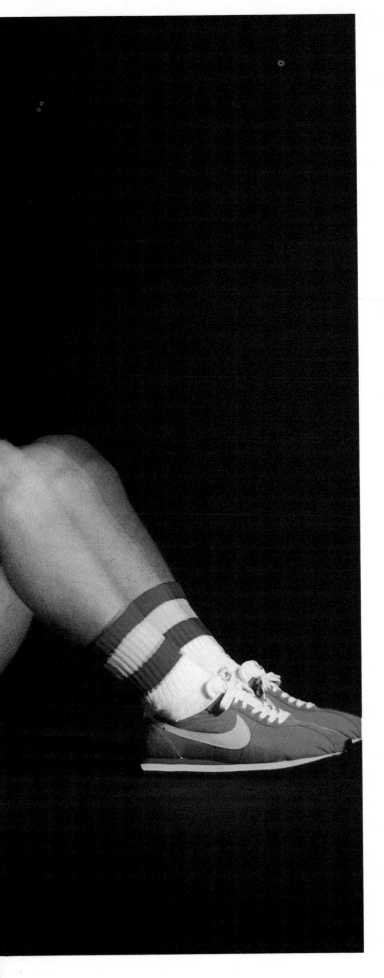

For Toning: Stretch and Flex

Good old-fashioned calisthenics can make you reach new heights in your quest for better health.

"**O**kay. Side-straddle-hop. Begin with feet together, arms at the sides. Ready, hup 2, hup 4, hup, hup. Now on your back, on your belly, on your back, and 8, and 9, and stop. Stand up, feet together, arms at the sides."

From the parade grounds at Fort Dix to the polished basketball court at Central High, this series of commands, usually shouted at the top of the instructor's voice, is a familiar one. Everyone who has ever taken a high school gym class or been in the military knows the litany well. In the military the drill instructor had you performing calisthenics well before the sun came up, and in gym the "coach," often a science teacher forced into emergency service, carried out his assigned job either right before or right after lunch.

The time was never right for regimented exercise and raw recruits and students alike performed the routines mechanically, with little knowledge of what the exercises were doing for them and no desire to find out. It was the way it was done that made it empty and boring, and everyone seemed to know it except the Pentagon and the board of education. It was just this kind of exercise and instruction that gave exercise in general, and calisthenics in particular, a bad name. That is, until calisthenic exercises were resurrected from obscurity in the 1970s.

In reality, those oft-repeated routines did a good job of limbering the body and increasing the heart rate. And the modern-day craze we know as aerobic dancing owes it all to basic calisthenics.

It's actually hard to determine where calisthenics stop and stretching and aerobics begin, because all the routines are active and stimulating for the system and they make use of many of the same motions. Proponents of stretching say that the jerkier, bouncier movements of calisthenics are hard on the muscles and joints and cause strains and soreness. They feel they have the answer because of the way stretching gradually limbers muscles and joints. Aerobics specialists say their method is best because it provides more exercise for the cardiovascular system. The calisthenics people fight back with the argument that their method is not only good for warming up, but is also aerobic.

But the controversy isn't really important. All of these methods of exercise accomplish the same end: an improvement in body tone, an increased heart rate, warmed muscles and, perhaps most important, flexibility.

STAY SUPPLE AND YOU'LL STAY YOUNGER

Why is flexibility crucial to health? To understand, we first have to understand just what flexibility is. Scientists define it as the "range of motion about a joint"—the maximum degree to which you can reach,

turn, twist, swing and bend. A baby, obviously, has a huge range; he thinks nothing of putting his foot in his mouth—a feat most adults can only manage by saying something foolish! That's because as we grow older, flexibility declines. We become tight, creaky, limited. Aging itself could be seen as a gradual decrease in flexibility.

In fact, many scientists believe that muscles deprived of exercise actually get shorter as we grow older. The longer these muscles are neglected, the shorter they will get, which is why being flexible is so important to health. By staying flexible we stay supple, loose—and young.

What are some of the most important facts researchers have found out about flexibility and exercise over the years?

- First of all, stretching *does* improve flexibility. A study at the University of Oregon showed that women who did routine stretching exercises became significantly more limber. And those who were considered in "average" shape at the begin-

No wonder they're called grunts! All U.S. military enlistees strain to get in shape to serve their country. Daily calisthenics and workouts became part of basic training after the Army found many unfit men signing up during World War I.

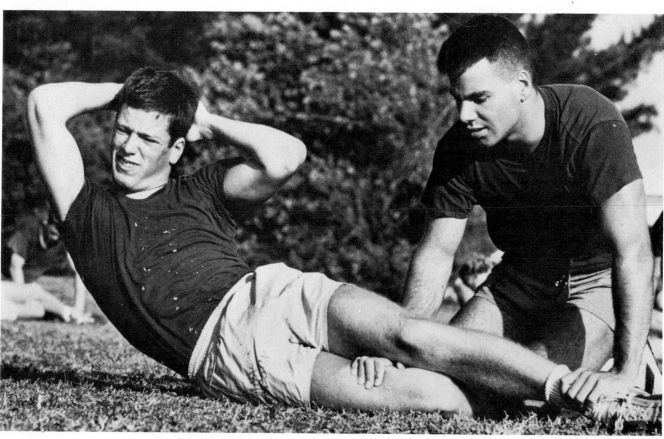

ning of the semester-long experiment made the greatest gains. A similar study at the University of Iowa found that women who took part in daily stretching exercises for three weeks improved substantially in virtually all flexibility tests.

- Warm-up exercises greatly improve mobility. Even a single preliminary movement, a toe touch, for example, results in a better score for that test. *Research Quarterly* reported a study involving 33 college men who were tested in the toe touch over a five-week period. Men who practiced the toe touch and other exercises before the test did considerably better than men who started cold. Another study with high school students and adults tested 20 joint movements and found that all 20 tests improved with warm-up. That's why athletes do stretching exercises before competing. They don't waste energy; they improve performance.

- There is no such thing as "normal" flexibility. This is because the range of natural movement varies so greatly from person to person. You can admire the person who can touch his toes with his elbows, but you don't have to be able to do it to be in the same physical shape.

- Flexibility is not the same throughout the body. Flexibility in one joint doesn't guarantee equal range of motion in other body parts. So you have to loosen up *all* of you, not just your back or legs.

- One of the oldest myths in the world of fitness and sports is that weight training causes a "muscle-bound" condition that limits an athlete's ability to move. Research has proven just the opposite. One study found that body builders who achieved international recognition in physique competitions and weight trainers who took part in weight-lifting events generally had greater flexibility than normal groups of 16-year-old boys. Another study found that in a speed test that required members of a university weight-lifting team and a control group of students to turn a crank at high speed, the weight lifters had arm movement speed equal to that of the other group.

THE FLEXIBILITY TEST

How flexible are you? Well, get on your feet and we'll find out. The idea of this little test is to find out how easily you can bend your body without any strain or pain. But be careful! If you haven't bent over without bending your knees in ten years, you can't expect to touch your toes. So don't force yourself. Here goes:

- Stand erect, with your hands at your sides and feet together. Keeping your knees locked, bend slowly from the waist. Stop when you begin to feel a tight resistance in the back of your legs or in your back. Are your fingers dangling somewhere around your knees? If so, you could use a little practice. Flexible men have no problem touching their toes. And women can even rest their palms on the floor.

- Now sit on the floor with your legs stretched out in front of you. Put an 8-inch-high book upright between your knees. Clasp your hands behind your head. Keeping your legs flat, lean forward until you feel that tell-tale strain. The really flexible person can touch the book with his forehead.

- Lie flat on your stomach with your hands clasped behind your neck and your feet touching the floor. How far can you raise your chin off the floor without straining? Don't be surprised if you can't raise it at all. The truly flexible person can get from 12 to 18 inches off the floor.

If you were an abysmal failure at any of the tests, read on. The exercises in this chapter are designed to improve your flexibility. If you follow them, you're bound to do much better when you get back to these tests a few months from now.

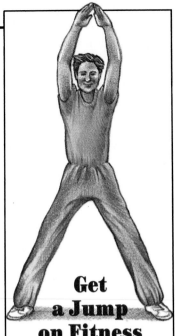

Get a Jump on Fitness

Jumping jacks may seem like child's play, but you'll get a good workout if you make them part of your daily exercise program. When it comes to calisthenics, jumping jacks are about the best. William B. Zuti, Ph.D., of the YMCA-USA, says that they work a variety of muscles, including those around the ribs, stomach and shoulders. They also tone some rarely used muscles like those along the insides of the thighs. It takes only a few minutes to really get your heart pumping. A reminder: Take it easy at first.

Daily Calisthenics

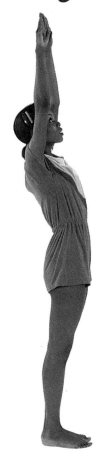

These exercises are simple and fun and they can be done with ease. A workout shouldn't take more than 15 or 20 minutes—less time than it takes many people to get out of bed. Do each exercise 3 times and move on to the next one. Slowly build your stamina until you can complete 3 circuits.

Standing Toe Touch

Stand with your feet a few inches apart and hands over your head. Bend at the hips, reaching for the ground as far as is comfortably possible. Hold for 10 seconds. Bend your knees to take the pressure off your back. Stand.

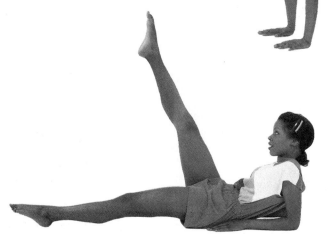

Pushups

Lie on the floor face down and balance your body on your toes and arms with the palms of your hands in line with your shoulders. Lower yourself until your elbows form a right angle and push back up. Or, if that's too difficult, balance your torso on your hands and knees and lower and raise yourself.

Leg Lifts

Sit on the floor with your legs straight and lean back until your elbows support you. Lift one leg as high as you comfortably can and hold it for a count of 10. Repeat with the other leg.

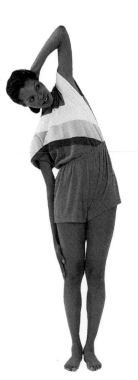

Side Lean

Stand erect and place your left palm flat behind your head. Put your right palm against your right thigh. Keep your legs together and reach down the right side toward your feet as far as is comfortable. Stand up again and repeat the exercise, switching arms and stretching the other side of the body. Don't strain or bounce to stretch farther.

Torso Swing

Stand erect and hold your arms out to your sides. Keep your feet straight and swing your body in a fluid movement to the right as far as is comfortable. Swing back to the left. Stretch the muscles in your torso with each swing.

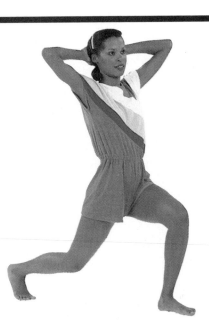

Squat Jump

Keep your feet 3 inches apart, with one foot directly behind the other and your knees slightly flexed. Clasp your hands behind your head and spring upward from the floor, reversing the position of your feet as you jump. Land in a semisquat position. Repeat for 30 seconds, reversing your feet each time.

Windmill

Stand with your knees bent slightly and your feet spread a shoulder width apart. Spread your arms out to the sides. Bend forward so that your left hand hits your right toe. Stand. Bend again until the right hand touches the left toe. Repeat.

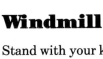

Jumping Jacks

Stand erect with your arms at your sides. Swing your arms above your head and clap once while jumping up slightly and spreading your feet. Then jump back to the starting position. Repeat. The jumps should be rhythmically paced.

Squat Thrust

Stand erect. Bend your knees and place your hands flat on the floor. Thrust your legs back until your body is straight. Return to squat. Stand.

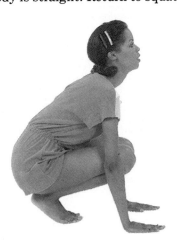

Wing Stretcher

Stand erect with your fists tight against your chest. Raise your elbows to shoulder height. Thrust your elbows backward vigorously and return. Repeat the movement, stretching your shoulders. Keep your head up when you thrust. Don't strain.

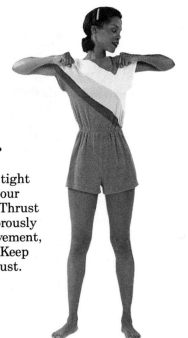

The Parcourse

One of the more enjoyable roads to fitness yet invented is the parcourse, a station-to-station fitness trail, usually through scenic woods or parks. Going through a parcourse is much like jogging and going to a gym at the same time. The idea is to jog from one station to the next, where a billboard will give you orders on exactly what exercise to do. The goal of the parcourse is twofold: it strengthens the heart and tones muscles. Check with your local parks and recreation departments or college to find the course nearest you.

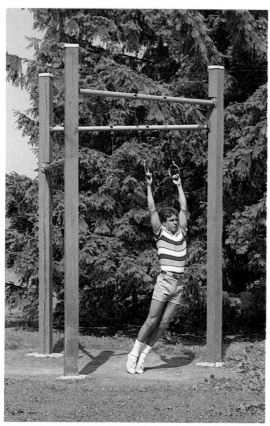

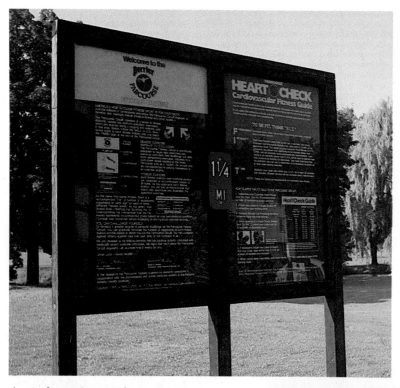

The circle body is a great way to stretch muscles. In fact, you're likely to find yourself stretching muscles you didn't even know you have! You must have a good grasp on the rings to get the full benefit of this exercise. Most courses have a set for different heights—even for half-pints.

At each station on the parcourse you'll get a complete set of instructions on how to carry out a specific exercise. At the start you'll do easy, warm-up routines. There are directions for 3 fitness levels: beginning, training and competition. Start low and aim high.

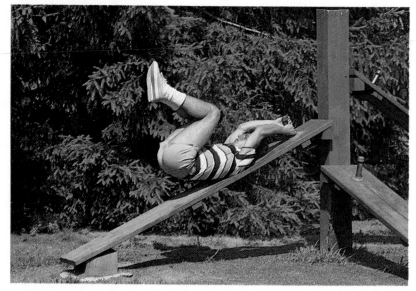

This is called the body curl and it's a tough one. The idea is to lie flat on the incline, grip the bar behind you and curl your body in a tuck position. Advanced parcourse users are told to do this exercise 10 times!

The toe touch is one of the exercises you'll be asked to do as you work your way through the beginning of the course. The idea is to limber up your muscles for bigger things to come.

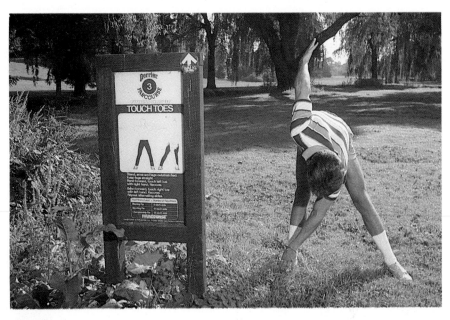

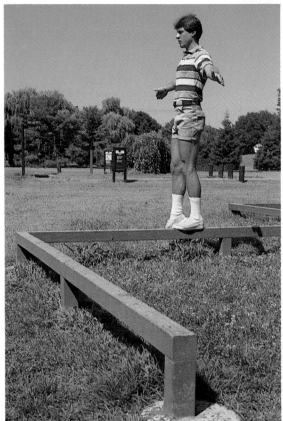

You probably haven't done anything like this since you were a kid. The log hop is a good way to get your heart pumping. But be careful, you'll have to jump quite a bit higher than you did when you played hopscotch.

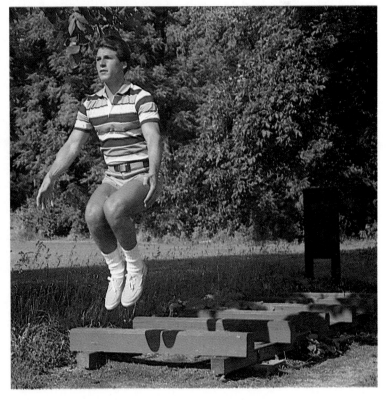

You needn't be an Olga Korbut to handle the balance beam on a parcourse. It usually comes at the end of the course and is intended as a fun way to cool down. You'll be asked to walk forward and backward along the beam. But it's not as easy as it looks. Some of you may find the backward walk a little tricky.

Daily Dozen

S tart out gently with these stretching exercises and work your muscles at their own pace. You will soon move more easily and your chances of suffering from sore joints and lower back pain will diminish. Take a deep breath after each stretch.

Arm Stretch

Hold one arm straight out from your side, level with the shoulder. Make an arc by raising your arm straight up, then lowering it to your side. Hold your arm out again. Swing it across your chest as far as is comfortable. Swing it toward your back as far as it will comfortably go. Now hold your arm straight in front of you, bending your elbow in a right angle with the palm toward the floor. Without moving your upper arm, move your forearm straight up and then straight down. Alternate arms.

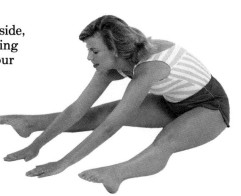

Sitting Stretch

Sit on the floor with your legs extended at least 6 to 10 inches apart. Bend forward with arms outstretched as far as you can and hold the position for 8 to 10 seconds. Do not strain or bounce.

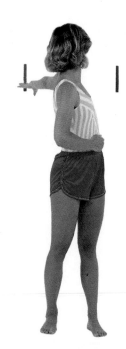

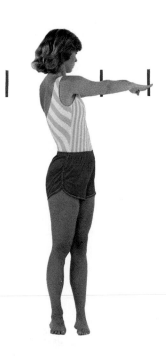

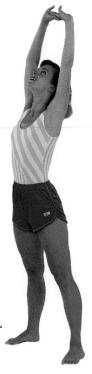

Sky Stretch

Stand with your feet spread apart. Clasp your hands high above your head. Lean your head back and look up. Stretch your shoulder muscles as if you were reaching for the sky. Hold for several seconds, or as long as is comfortable. Relax. Repeat 2 to 4 times.

Side Stretch

Make 3 imaginary marks at shoulder height on a wall at about 1-foot intervals. Stand with your back to the wall, an arm's length away. Extend one arm and twist your body, touching each mark with your hand. Reach as far as possible. Change sides and repeat.

Double Stretch

Using the same marks as for the side stretch, stand 3 feet from the wall. With your back to the wall and your feet about 2 feet apart, bend and touch the floor. Straighten up. Twist your body and touch the marks on the wall. Return to starting position and repeat, this time twisting to the other side.

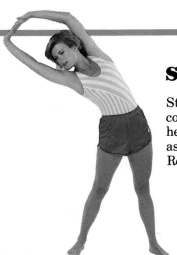

Side Stretch

Stand straight with your legs spread comfortably. Clasp your hands above your head. Lean from the waist to the right as far as is comfortable without moving your hip. Repeat, leaning to the left.

Floor Touch

Stand erect with your legs spread. Bring your hands together in front of you. Bend at the waist and try to touch the floor. Don't strain! Hold for 10 seconds. Return to starting position and repeat.

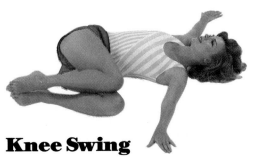

Leg Arc

Stand straight with your arms at your sides. In one continuous motion, swing your leg straight out to one side. Swing it back across your other leg as far as comfortably possible. Return to starting position and repeat with the other leg.

Knee Swing

Lie on your back with your arms outstretched and palms down. Keeping your ankles together, raise your knees to your chest and roll your knees to touch the floor, first on one side, then the other. Keep your hands and shoulders firmly on the floor. Repeat 15 to 30 times.

Pedal Stretch

Lie on your right side with your head resting on your outstretched arm and the palm of your left hand on the floor in front of your chest. Raise your legs slightly off the floor and pedal for 10 seconds as if you were riding a bicycle. Switch sides and repeat.

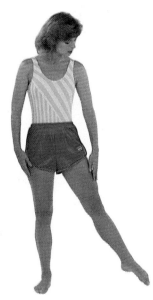

Horizontal Leg Stretch

Lie on your back with both legs outstretched. Bend your right knee and raise it until your foot is a few inches off the floor. Keeping your hips straight, slide your left leg to the left along the floor. Slide it back and lower the other leg. Repeat the exercise, alternating legs.

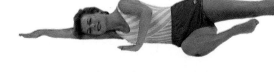

Leg Extension

Lie on your back with one knee bent and your foot on the floor. Slowly raise the other leg to a vertical position, or as far as is comfortably possible. Lower it slowly. Repeat with the other leg.

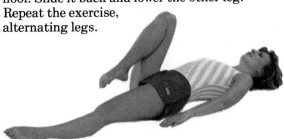

Posture Exercises

If you have ever watched a great runner, you have probably noticed that his or her running seems almost effortless, even though every muscle in the body is being used to its capacity. The head is high and steady, the back is straight and the arms pump directly forward and back. Every movement is efficient. Even when near exhaustion, the great runners maintain this efficiency of movement. This style of running, though it doesn't seem like it, is the result of good posture and body awareness. All extra movements —flapping hands, flailing arms, heels kicked too high, excessive trunk movement—waste energy.

What is normally referred to as posture is merely the relationship of various parts of the body to each other. Though most people think posture is only the way we stand, it really is the way we carry ourselves at all times, whether standing, sitting, or lying down.

Unfortunately, there are more people with bad posture than with good. The bad back, protruding stomach and sagging shoulders are glaring, telltale signs of bad posture that can be detected by the most casual observer. In fact, as you read these words, you are probably sitting in a slumped position in a chair that is too soft to give support to your back.

Now get in front of the mirror and we'll tell you the *right* way to carry yourself.

Stand erect, keeping your body firm, yet flexible. Relax. Look straight ahead and distribute your weight evenly on the ball of each foot—not the toes or heel. You should be able to raise your heels without leaning forward.

Slightly tilt your lower pelvis forward and upward. Imagine that you're holding a coin between your buttocks and you'll feel them tightening (don't bend your knees). As you shift into position, your buttocks should tuck in and the small of the back—the lumbar curve—should flatten into a slight arc.

Hold your chest high. As you raise your chest, your shoulders naturally roll back and your stomach pulls in.

Your goal is good vertical

Problems of Poor Posture

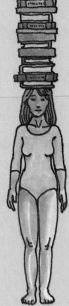

Many slouchers accept posture-related problems as a fact of life. And there are plenty of problems to accept.

The most common result of poor posture is lower back pain, and back pain afflicts at least 8 of 10 Americans in their lifetime. When your posture is bad, the natural curves in your spine are exaggerated. These curves pick up your body's weight, which, according to Leon Root, M.D., author of *Oh, My Aching Back*, "causes excessive wear and tear earlier than normal in the spine's life." Some doctors recommend building up your abdominal muscles so they'll take pressure off the back.

Poor posture can also cause neckaches and headaches. When you work with your head hunched forward or sleep with a pile of pillows under your head, your neck muscles strain to keep your head erect. This fatigue can spread upward, causing your head to ache.

Bad posture can get worse as you get older, but it's never too late to correct it. Just keep in mind that the longer you neglect it, the more effort you'll need to reverse it.

alignment. That is, you should be able to drop an imaginary plumb line from just behind the ear, through the shoulder and the sacrum (the last bone of the spine and part of the pelvis), behind the hip and the knee and through the ankle.

Although it sounds like quite a goal—connecting all those bones—there are only three maneuvers to remember. Stand erect. Tilt your pelvis. Raise your chest. Everything else takes care of itself and falls naturally into place.

Don't be discouraged if you find yourself twisting like a go-go dancer in front of the mirror while trying to align your body. Chances are your body is accustomed to being "out of line," and good posture may seem uncomfortable or unnatural at first.

Good posture is a skill, just like playing a musical instrument or riding a bicycle. And like other skills, it will improve steadily with practice. The exercises shown here are designed to change your bad posture into perfect posture.

Shoulder Stretch

Stand as straight as possible and clasp your hands behind your head. Pull your elbows up and back as far as possible and hold for 3 seconds. Relax and repeat.

Leg Out

Stand erect with your hands clasped behind your head. Get up on your toes and then swing one leg forward, keeping it straight and the toes pointed down. Return to the starting position and repeat with the other leg.

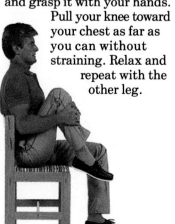

Bend

Stand straight with your feet together and clasp your hands behind your back, keeping your arms extended. Then bend over at the waist and raise your clasped hands as high as you can above your shoulders. Return to the starting position and repeat.

Sit Stretch I

Sit with your back straight against a chair and put your feet flat on the floor. Fold your arms across the top of your head. Touch your elbows with your fingers. Relax and repeat.

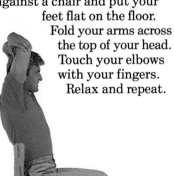

Sit Stretch II

Sit with your back straight against a chair. Put your arms behind the chair, clasp your forearms and pull your shoulders back. Relax and repeat.

Knee Hold

Sit with your back straight against a chair and your feet flat on the floor. Lift one knee and grasp it with your hands. Pull your knee toward your chest as far as you can without straining. Relax and repeat with the other leg.

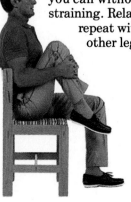

6

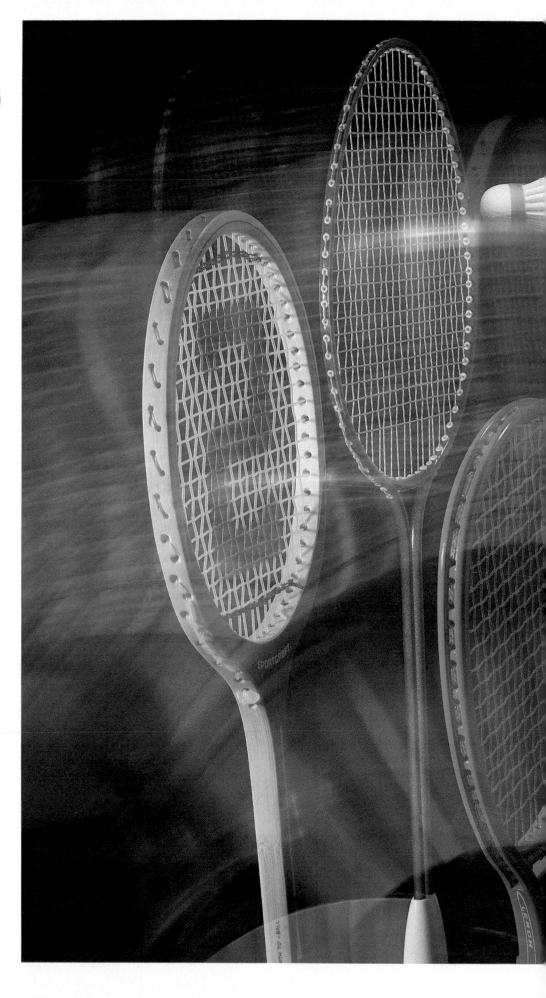

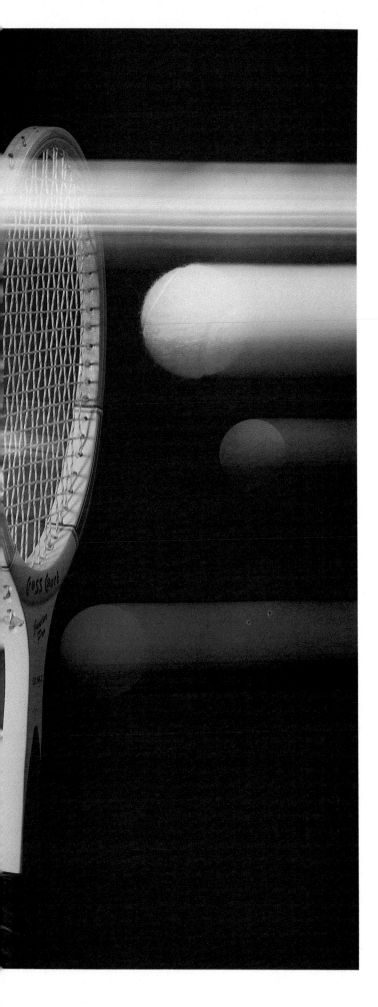

Fitness with Fun

Recreational sports are the best way to work your active life into your social life.

Of course you really want to be in top physical condition. Who doesn't? After all, everyone knows that a healthy life is a happier life. And there's something particularly pleasing, an inner satisfaction, that comes with fitness—when a glance in the mirror discloses no unwelcome bulges, when you can bound to the top of the stairs without nearing collapse, when friends and acquaintances guess your age and they always guess too low.

But you say there's a problem. You find the repetitious rigors of running somewhat repulsive, the silent strokes of swimming too stifling, the work of weight lifting too wearisome. Well, take heart. There's a way around this problem, a way to mix fitness with fun.

Welcome to the world of recreational sports!

History does not tell us who thought up the first physically active game, or what it was. But we would not be surprised to learn that the idea came from a person who managed only to mutter "Ugh!" when confronted with the idea that the road to fitness was pockmarked with potholes of pain, loneliness and boredom.

Today, with a little searching, anybody can find a game to suit his or her pleasure and particular skills, a game that will provide those very same health benefits that are so excruciatingly acquired by the more zealous fitness buffs. From racquetball to roller skating, the list of activities that build strength, enhance cardiovascular efficiency and help to control weight is almost endless. Best of all, properly chosen, the games that people play have that all-important common ingredient—fun.

Naturally, you must choose a sport that will hold your interest, one that is in concert with your personal skills. There is a direct relationship between your level of competence and the amount of benefit you get. Simply stated, the better you get at your favorite sports, the more they will do for you—and the more fun you will have!

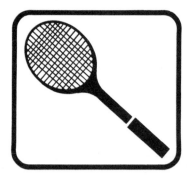

Tennis

There are at least 25 million tennis players in the United States —that alone ought to tell you whether the game is any fun.

One reason that may account for its phenomenal success is that tennis is an athletic game in which men and women can compete recreationally. But anyone who has played the game knows that there also is a special satisfaction to a service ace, an overhead smash or a well-executed shot that catches an opponent off guard.

Naturally, the beginning tennis player will not experience all of the joys of the game immediately. Tennis is a game that requires patience, concentration and lots of practice. That's why it is advisable to take a few lessons (group lessons are fine) or play with someone of equal ability or someone who's a little better than yourself. It's not necessary to be an expert to enjoy the game, but it gets to be more and more fun as you sharpen your skills.

Importantly, as you get better at it, the game will get better for you.

One study, involving 50 middle-aged adults whose only form of exercise was playing tennis approximately 10 hours a week, was conducted by doctors at Stanford University. They found that the tennis players showed better-than-average pulse rate, blood pressure and proportion of body fat.

The researchers cautioned that such a small study could not prove conclusively that tennis was the reason for the superior condition of the subjects, but other expert opinions add weight to that theory. Fitness experts David Shepro, Ph.D., and Howard Knuttgen, Ph.D., maintain that "tennis played by skilled players capable of extended rallies can make a meaningful, although not great, contribution to the cardiovascular system."

So the evidence is mounting that tennis can be quite good for you. Millions already know how enjoyable it can be. Instead of just batting the breeze about exercise, why not try batting a tennis ball around sometime soon?

It's not who wins, but how you play the game that counts if you want to mix your love of tennis with your need for exercise. The only way to make a tennis game a truly aerobic workout is to pick a partner who can challenge your own ability. That also means running—not meandering—around the court to retrieve stray balls.

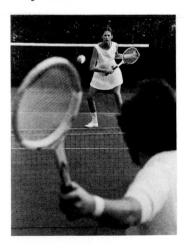

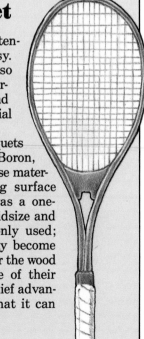

Choosing a Racquet

It used to be that choosing a tennis racquet was relatively easy. They all were made of wood, so the player had only to determine the optimum grip size and racquet weight, and the material of the strings.

Now, however, there are racquets made of aluminum, fiberglass, Boron, graphite or any combination of these materials. Even the size of the hitting surface varies. While in the past there was a one-size-only racquet, there are now midsize and oversize racquets that are commonly used; some say the smaller racquets may become obsolete. Top players generally prefer the wood and composition racquets because of their ability to absorb vibrations. The chief advantage of an aluminum racquet is that it can provide more power.

The Basic Strokes

Forehand Drive. Begin with a high backswing as you step forward. Move your shoulders and hips sideways toward the ball as you complete the backswing. Then, swing the racquet through as you step into the stroke, making contact with the ball off your front foot. (Your weight is moving forward.) Follow through with your knees still bent from your position when you made contact with the ball.

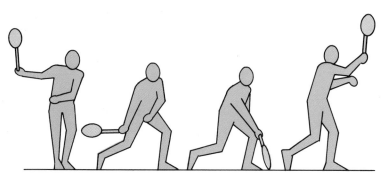

Backhand Drive. Using your left hand to draw the racquet back, turn your shoulders, arms and racquet together and step forward. With your eye on the ball, draw the racquet through and hit the ball in front of your front foot. With the racquet parallel to the ground and your body sideways to the net, keep your arm straight and wrist locked. Follow through with your knees bent and your opposite arm extended for balance.

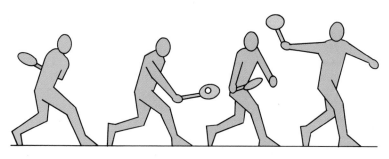

Forehand Volley. The forehand volley can be used to execute a shot on the run. As the body pivots, the left arm helps with balance.

Backhand Volley. Unlike a backhand drive, a backhand volley is used to return the ball before it hits the ground. Hit the ball out front, keeping your wrist firm and your weight on the balls of your feet. You can use your opposite hand to guide the racquet back.

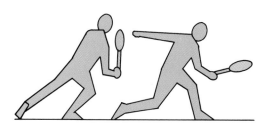

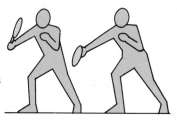

The Service. With your weight forward and the racquet head up, let both arms fall and transfer your weight to your back foot. Throw the ball lightly in the air, swinging the racquet back and up and putting your body into a sideways turn. Swing the racquet up behind your head, then directly overhead to smack the ball. Contact should be made as your shoulders come parallel to the net. Finally, let your weight carry you forward as you complete the swing by bringing the racquet across your body.

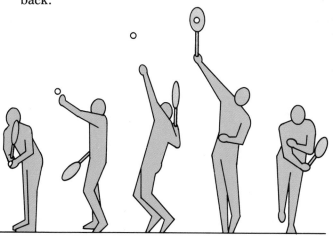

Racquetball

I t's relatively easy to learn, it's fun to play, it's equally rewarding to men and women and it's great exercise. "It" is racquetball, a sport that traces its ancestry to both handball and tennis.

You can thank Joseph G. Sobek, a New York and Connecticut instructor of squash and tennis, for this game. In the 1950s, Sobek began playing handball for enjoyment. He soon realized that the sport was too difficult and painful for most people, since it involved slugging a hard rubber ball against the walls of an enclosed court with unpadded gloves. But he also obviously saw great potential in the concept of the game, a game in which two to four players carom shots off the walls and ceiling of a 20-foot by 40-foot court in an attempt to get the ball beyond the opponent's reach.

So Sobek, always the innovator, got together with friends and they played essentially the same game with one difference—they used a paddle instead of their hands. Sobek continued experiments until he came up with a stubby stringed racquet—a kind of sawed-off tennis racquet—and a rubber ball with the proper amount of bounce. Racquetball, as we know it today, was here.

Fitness researchers have found that this enjoyable game can provide important health benefits. When played two or three times a week it promotes muscle development, hand/eye coordination and flexibility. It also can provide excellent aerobic exercise if both players are fairly competent, of like ability and sufficiently motivated to keep the game moving at a fast clip.

Then there's the added psychological benefit—the satisfaction of hitting hard, really sending the ball careening around the court. For the stress-filled executive, this can be a socially acceptable way of letting go of aggression.

Since racquetball involves quick starts and stops, plus a lot of stretching and bending, it should be preceded by a warm-up period and followed by a cool-down of approximately 5 minutes each. This will prevent overtaxing of the heart and also help to avoid tears and pulls.

Injuries are relatively minor in racquetball, generally resulting from turning an ankle or getting hit accidentally by the opponent's racquet. The soft rubber ball will not cause any serious damage, despite its great speed, unless it should hit a person in the eye. This is why wearing eye protectors or shatterproof glasses is advisable.

Racquetball has great appeal for young and old, male and female, skilled and unskilled. It can be a wise choice for anyone who wants to achieve fitness in a way that is thoroughly enjoyable.

Racquetball can be a good aerobic workout—but only if you work up a lot of steam and get your body moving along with the ball. Goggles are a must, too. You're only courting trouble without them.

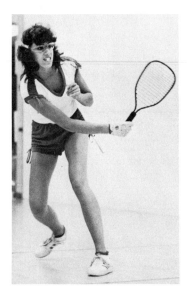

A Sport in Big Demand

From its start in the 1950s, racquetball has grown into a game that boasts more than 10 million players, and it shows no sign of slowing down.

In fact, its popularity has increased so rapidly, particularly in the last 15 years, that there is a demand for courts that still hasn't been met. Estimates place the number of court clubs in existence at over 1,600 and new ones continue to be built. Interest in it is so keen that there are plans to include it in the Pan-American Games.

The Basic Strokes

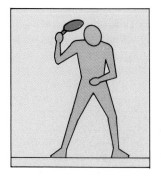 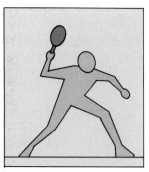 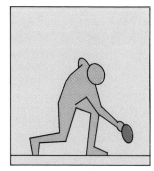 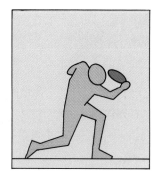

Basic Forehand Stroke. Get behind the ball and lift the racquet to head height, with your wrist cocked back. Balancing on the balls of your feet, stride forward with your front foot and swing evenly into the stroke, bending your knees and waist to reach the ball. Let the elbow lead the stroke, powered by the rotation of your hip and shoulders. Just before impact, bring your lower arm through and snap your wrist. Meet the ball at knee height as your weight comes forward. Follow through close to your body.

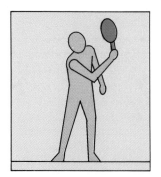 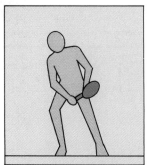 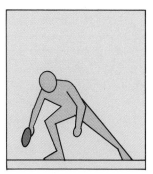 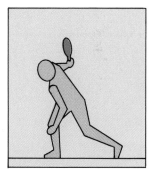

Basic Backhand Stroke. On the backswing, take your weight back onto your back foot, with hips turned away and lead shoulder tucked in. Begin the stroke with wrist uncocked. Leaning forward, let your hips and elbow lead into the stroke. Take a shorter stride than for the forehand swing but bend more to keep your racquet parallel to the floor. Meet the ball just in front of your front foot. Snap the wrist from uncocked to cocked, and follow through with care.

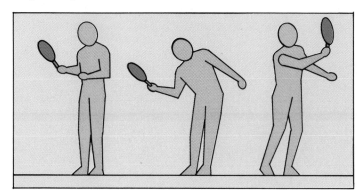 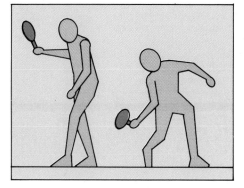

"Garbage" Service. The best serve is aimed at the opponent's backhand in order to get a weak return. The "garbage" service is the most frequently used; when it is executed properly, the ball will bounce back to touch the floor about 3 feet behind the short line, then bounce again before dying in the rear corner. To serve, bounce the ball to rebound at waist or chest height, then hit the ball at the peak of its bounce with a pushing motion. Add some spin, too.

Drive Service. The short service comes from off center, rebounding to touch the floor just past the short line. The long serve comes from the center and rebounds before going low to the rear corner. Drop the ball so it returns to calf or knee height by your front foot as you step into the stroke. Hit it at the peak of its bounce with a forehand stroke.

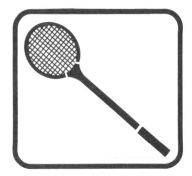

Squash

Nobody knows for sure just how the game of squash came to be. One theory says that it was devised by inmates of a London prison as a form of indoor recreation. Another says it was invented by students at an English school and got its name from the sound of the ball hitting the wall.

Although its name certainly gives no indication, squash is another of the indoor racquet games. Although it is played on a smaller court, employs a different type of racquet and ball and is scored differently, it is not unlike racquetball. Stated simply, the players bat the ball around an enclosed court until somebody is unable to return a shot.

The smallish court and the badmintonlike racquet tend to belie the amount of energy required to play an accomplished game of squash. But, one study has shown that an intensive game of squash can be every bit as aerobic as running. Although the average length of a rally may be less than 10 seconds, if you play with a partner of equal ability and fitness level you'll get a good cardiovascular workout.

Squash has never really attained the popularity of racquetball, one reason being that there are not nearly as many courts. But if you live near a court, you would do well to investigate the pleasures—and benefits—it offers.

Maybe it's because of its snob appeal, but whatever the real reason, squash has never captured the population at large as a popular racquet sport. Actually, it's not much different from racquetball, either in the way it's played or in the benefits it gives the body.

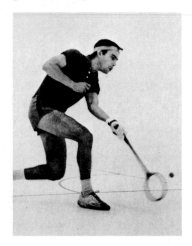

The Basic Strokes

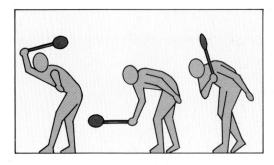

Forehand and Backhand Drives. Turning to the side wall, backswing with your elbow bent and wrist cocked. (The racquet is angled behind your head.) Lead in with your elbow, straightening it before impact. Bend your back and knees so that the racquet is parallel to the floor. With weight forward, meet the ball at the peak of its bounce, level with your front foot. Keep your racquet face open and wrist cocked. Follow through upward, close to your body, wrist cocked, elbow bent.

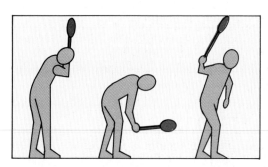

Lob Service. This serve should strike the front wall about center court, nearer the out-of-court line than the cut line. It returns as a lob, crossing the other service box, touching high on the side wall, then dropping to the floor and bouncing to the back corner.

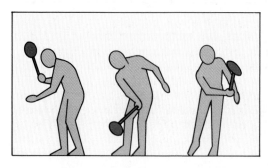

Table Tennis

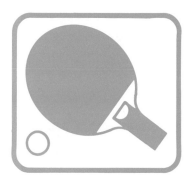

The game of table tennis has come a long way since the late 1800s when, according to the most popular theory, it was started by English army officers stationed in India. Looking for recreation, they carved champagne corks into balls and hit them back and forth across books piled in the center of a dining room table.

The game took an important step forward about 1890 when James Gibb, founder of the Amateur Athletic Association in England, purchased celluloid balls on a business trip to the United States and introduced them to the game when he returned home. It was Gibb who coined the game's other name, Ping-Pong, because of the sound the ball made when hitting the paddle and then the table.

Today, with modern equipment and a standardized set of rules, the game is popular in at least 120 countries and may be the most widely played of all sports, even eclipsing soccer.

Played at its most competitive level, table tennis can be very demanding, requiring extensive physical conditioning. But enjoyed as a recreational sport, it does not contribute significantly to increased strength or aerobic fitness. What it does do is improve hand/eye coordination and keep the reflexes working at peak levels. Importantly, it also is a game that can be started and enjoyed by people of all ages.

Players well into their senior years can maintain very credible levels of competition. Persons confined to wheelchairs can enjoy it, too. It's also easy to take up and inexpensive, and it can be played year-round, all of which add to the game's appeal.

The Basic Strokes

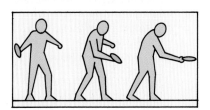

Backhand Push. Shift your weight forward, striking the ball at the peak of the bounce. Follow through with your arm until it is straight, lifting the ball.

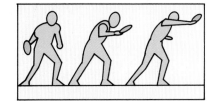

Forehand Flat Attack. This stroke is like the backhand, but your left hip is toward the table. More body movement is required.

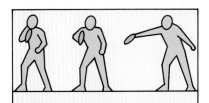

Forehand Push. Begin with your weight on your right foot, with your left shoulder and foot forward. Drop your right shoulder as your weight moves forward to strike the ball; follow through with your arm low.

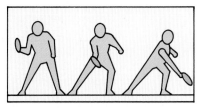

Backspin Chop. This stroke is almost vertical, starting high and ending low so the paddle chops downward against the ball. Play close to the table with your body turned only half away, or at a distance with your body sideways.

Table tennis, or Ping-Pong, as we more fondly call it, is one of those games you play when you feel like batting something about in the family recreation room. But don't think of it as one step more active than watching TV. When actively pursued, table tennis can give you a good physical workout.

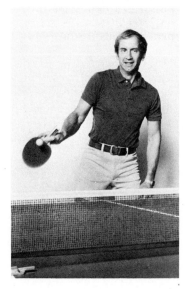

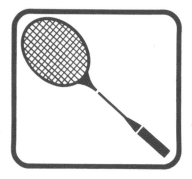

Badminton

There are two features of badminton that make it a great racquet sport for the beginner.

One is the racquet, which is so light that even young children can easily swing it. The second is the shuttlecock, or bird, as it is commonly called, which consists of feathers stuck in a cork base. No matter how hard the bird is hit, the feathers eventually catch the air and it begins a gentle descent to the ground. As the result of these features, it is possible for novices to keep rallies going the first time they play the game.

Another plus for the game is that the only other requirements are a net and a 20-foot by 44-foot space. Therefore, it can be played outdoors or indoors.

In terms of exercise, badminton provides the average player with muscle fitness from stretching and aerobic fitness from the running that is required to keep the bird in play. On the other hand, expert-level badminton requires superior conditioning as well as tremendous cunning. A champion can hit the shuttlecock at 100 miles per hour, or turn it in midstroke, in some totally unexpected direction.

The exact origin of badminton is unknown. One version claims it is an outgrowth of the ancient children's game of battledore and shuttlecock. It began to take its modern shape in the 1860s at the estate of the Duke of Beaufort in Badminton, England, which explains how it got its name.

Today the game remains a minority sport, although there is an International Badminton Federation which has links with more than 70 countries; in some of them—such as Denmark, Malaya, Thailand and Indonesia—it is a major national sport. Badminton is easy to learn and can be played almost anywhere, making it an excellent choice for families, neighbors or other groups who want to enjoy keeping fit.

Unlike its more strenuous cousins, badminton is a racquet sport that's welcome just about anywhere. Consider making the carry-it-with-you game part of your fitness regimen for those listless days at the park, the beach or on a family outing when a bit of spontaneous exercise is in order. And don't let the ease of the game fool you. Taken seriously, an airborne "bird" can keep you on your toes more than you think.

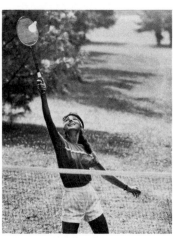

Buying the Best

Badminton racquet strings are made of either nylon or gut, with gut now used almost exclusively in the expensive racquets preferred by expert players. This is slowly changing, though, because the top-quality gut is being taken for medical sutures. A cheap outdoor badminton set, which includes 4 racquets, costs as little as $10 to $15. A single top-quality racquet used for tournament play can cost as much as $75.

Badminton racquets generally are made of tubular metal, usually steel. But graphite is becoming an increasingly popular material.

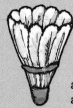

The shuttlecock, or bird, has a cork base and feathers, usually from a goose. However, plastic and nylon birds are now made for recreational use.

All good badminton racquets have leather grips. Although racquets are a standard size, the grip area differs in length, depending on the manufacturer. An advantage of leather is that it absorbs moisture well and does not slip in the hand. Interestingly, the manufacture of quality badminton racquets is pretty much the exclusive province of Taiwan and England.

Handball

Handball is not a game for the faint of heart. It is so physically demanding and difficult to master that it is generally taken up by well-conditioned athletes who are already accomplished in other sports. Some fitness experts believe that handball requires the use of more muscles than any other sport except swimming.

The game dates back to ancient Egypt, when players exchanged shots by smacking a crude ball against a single wall. Today, in the United States, the game in its most popular form is played in an enclosed court 40 feet long, 20 feet wide and 20 feet high.

What makes handball such a tough game initially is that it involves smacking a golf-ball-size hard rubber ball against the walls and ceiling with both hands. Contact with the ball is painful until the hands are toughened and attempting to play skillfully with the weak hand can be extremely frustrating. With the tremendous speed and spin the ball generates, handball requires lightning-fast starts and stops and lots of sudden bending and stretching. It tones arm and leg muscles, promotes weight loss and is a tremendous game for developing and maintaining cardiovascular fitness.

Skilled players recommend a conditioning program before the game is even started. While handball is excellent for maintaining physical fitness, it also is an extremely "mental" game. At all levels, it involves outguessing the opponent's next move.

Because of its extreme difficulty, handball is enjoyed mostly by a fraternity of athletically inclined enthusiasts who get their recreational pleasure from strenuously competitive physical activity.

Looking for a Racquet Sport?

With racquet in hand there seems no end to the games you can play. Here are a few more choices. Or, you can make up your own.

Platform Tennis

 The court on which platform tennis is played looks just like a regulation tennis court, only it is one-third the size and is enclosed by a 12-foot-high wire screen. Using a wooden paddle and sponge rubber ball, it follows the same rules as tennis, with 2 exceptions. First, the ball may be played as it rebounds off the screen. This difference makes it easier to keep the ball in play, even for a novice. Also, only 1 serve is allowed, so that power hitters do not have the advantage.

Paddleball

 A spinoff from handball, paddleball is played against 1, 3 or 4 walls with wooden paddles of various shapes and grip sizes. A soft, rather than hard, rubber ball is used. From its simple beginning, it has become a sophisticated game with angle shots and a variety of strokes.

Kadima

 You may have seen it often—2 people with paddles batting a ball back and forth on the beach. The game they were playing is Kadima. Also known as Smash-ball, this game has no strict rules. The idea, simply, is to keep volleying the ball. Kadima involves minimal running, but there is lots of stretching and it's good for hand/eye coordination.

Handball is a recreational sport, but let the person beware who dares step onto the court without being in good physical shape! Because it requires lightning reflexes, a strong (and hardened) hand and great physical energy, it's a sport best left to only conditioned athletes.

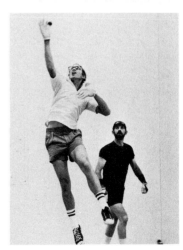

Downhill Skiing

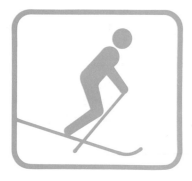

A crisp winter day with a layer of freshly fallen snow beckons you to the slopes for an exhilarating day of downhill skiing. What a thrill for millions of Americans who get to know the feeling each winter!

But this sport, which began thousands of years ago as transportation, not recreation, should not be entered into lightly. In fact, much of the fitness that the enthusiastic skier enjoys should be acquired long before that first downhill run.

Conditioning for skiing is really overall conditioning, involving the building of endurance, muscular strength, flexibility, agility, coordination and balance. Even when fit, skiers should warm up carefully before attacking the slopes.

The primary reason for all the emphasis on conditioning is, of course, to avoid injury. The sport puts unusual strain on the musculature, especially in the lower body. Muscle tears and broken bones are the unhappy result for thousands each year. For the same reason, equipment should be chosen carefully. Modern skis, bindings and boots are designed to minimize injuries during those inevitable spills that beginners, and even accomplished skiers, will take.

Skiing is a relatively expensive sport that requires a significant investment in equipment and clothing, plus money for transportation and the use of the many slopes that dot the colder regions of the country. But properly prepared for, it is recreation that promotes fitness and is thoroughly enjoyable to people of all ages.

From the Alpine resorts of Switzerland to the beautiful Colorado ranges of Aspen, nothing can quite reach the heights of downhill skiing when it comes to glamorous exercise. But any smart skier will get into shape *before* hitting the slopes. It's one of those sports that will help keep you in shape, rather than get you in shape.

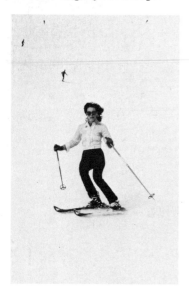

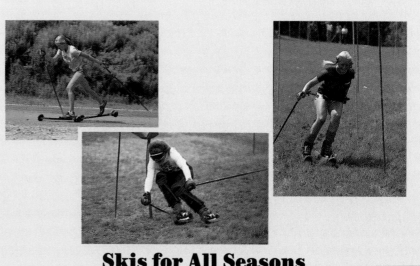

Skis for All Seasons

So, who needs snow? There are ways for ski buffs to stay happy and on a pair of skis all year long. Not only is it a unique way to enjoy the sport, it's also a great way to keep in shape. The "roller skis" at top left are cousins of the standard cross-country models but have rubber tires that enable the skier to slide over level, paved surfaces with the same stride used with the snow variety. Downhill ski fans can don regular ski boots and slip on a pair of "grass skis," shown center and right, with tractor-type treads. The pace on grass is a little slower than on snow. In fact, for beginners, this can be an easy way to learn the sport.

Ice Skating

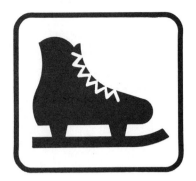

It wasn't too long ago that ice skating was pretty much a regional and seasonal form of recreation. But with a growth in popularity and the subsequent burgeoning of indoor rinks, ice skating has become an accessible sport all across the country.

In fact, there are an estimated 15 million ice skaters in the United States, and California is one of the states with the most devotees.

If you think of ice skating as a serene sport in which you slide effortlessly across a mirrorlike surface, you are in for a surprise. Skating offers aerobic benefit and leg strengthening comparable to jogging—without putting wear and tear on the knees. Because of the necessary arm motion, it actually exceeds jogging in contributing to upper body strength.

One feature of ice skating that makes it stand apart from other forms of recreation is that it can be enjoyed alone, in pairs or in groups.

It can be as pleasurable to the novice as to highly trained professional figure skaters and hockey players. However, experts do recommend one thing: Everyone taking up skating should begin on figure skates instead of hockey skates. This is because the blade is wider and the skate shoe is closer to the ground, making that initial struggle for balance an easier chore.

To many people, competitive figure skating—which began in 1926—is one of the most beautiful sports, on a par with ballet. At that level, it is also one of the most physically demanding, requiring the agility of a gymnast, the stamina of a long-distance runner and, of course, the grace of a dancer. Only a few take ice skating to that level. But it matters not, because it offers bountiful rewards in pleasure and good health at all levels.

Caring for Your Skates

A good pair of ice skates has a genuine leather shoe and an adjustable steel blade that holds its edge, and will last a long time with only a minimum of care. Experts recommend that those who skate on a pond should sharpen their skates after 5 to 10 uses. Rink skaters should sharpen theirs more frequently. Good polish will keep the shoe in good condition, but the tongue should be pulled out after use to promote drying. Skates should not be stored in the rubber guards that are used for walking off the ice because the blades tend to "sweat" in hot weather. Instead, they should be kept in terry cloth booties.

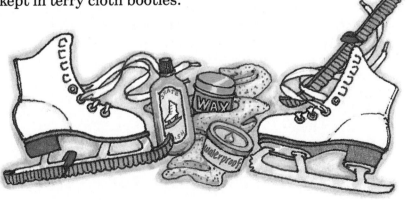

You may need the gentle grace of a ballerina to copy the delicate maneuvers of a top-notch ice skater. But if skating for fun and exercise is your sole goal, all you need to depend on is your trusty balance and coordination. Good physical conditioning will be your reward.

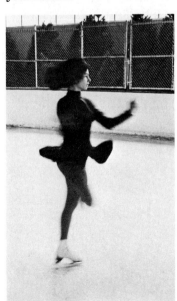

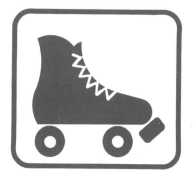

Roller Skating

You probably think of roller skating as kid's stuff. It is that, but it's also a whole lot more. It's a great social activity, it's terrific exercise and it's even a practical form of transportation.

Back in the mid-1600s, when wooden spools were nailed to strips of wood and attached to shoes, probably no one realized what a popular activity roller skating would become. And with good reason. Those early skates were practically unmanageable. It took an American, James Leonard Plimpton, to solve the problem in 1863 with a controllable, four-wheeled "rocking skate" that was the forerunner of the modern skate.

From that time on, roller skating, like roller coaster riding, has had its ups and downs, swinging from periods of great popularity to times of relative disuse. Most recently, following the development of smoother, faster and more comfortable polyurethane wheels in the 1960s, roller skating soared to a popularity it enjoys to this day. With the widespread use of roller skates outdoors as well as in skating rinks, it was only a matter of time until the health experts checked to see what fitness benefits skating had to offer.

Researchers from the University of California at Los Angeles, in a ten-week study of untrained adult skaters, found that roller skating is an excellent form of aerobic exercise. Allen Selner, D.P.M., director of sports medicine for the U.S. Amateur Confederation of Roller Skating and leader of the study, reports research "confirmed that roller skating is equivalent to jogging in terms of its health benefits—caloric consumption, reduction of body fat and leg strength development." And, to top it off, more than 90 percent of the skaters showed a significant reduction in stress and anxiety.

The gain in skating's popularity has spawned a whole range of rolling activities—skate dancing, skate racing, stunt skating, roller derbies and even a skate-to-work movement. If you haven't found yourself a life sport, you might just lace yourself into a comfortable pair of skates and glide to new-found health.

If you haven't laced up a pair of roller skates since you were a child, it may be time to do so again. The power you put behind those wheels is a great form of aerobic exercise. And besides, it'll make you feel, well, like a kid again!

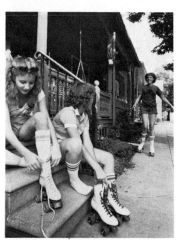

On a Roll? Here's How to Stop

There's more to roller skating than simply zooming along. You must be able to stop, too. If you're rolling backward, the problem is minimal. Just drag the rubber stop at the front of the skating shoe along the skating surface. Traveling forward is a different matter. Beginners usually are taught to balance their weight on one skate and drag the other one along behind it. The experienced skater can slow himself in much the same manner as a skier, either by snowplowing or by quickly changing the direction of the skates.

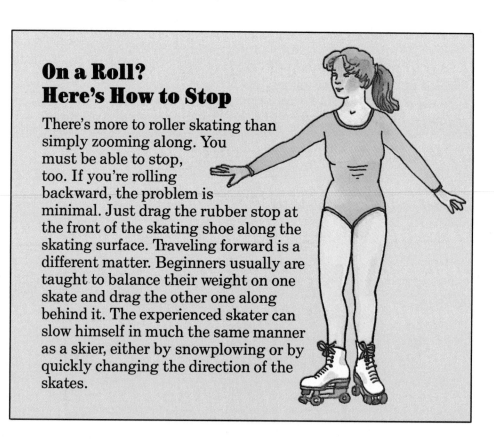

Hiking

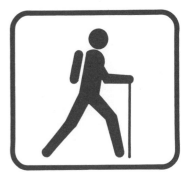

Here's an exercise that's inexpensive, readily available, healthful for young and old and simple. It's hiking. And everyone can do it—if you can walk, you can hike.

Hiking can open a whole new world, taking you to nature's most beautiful and awesome nooks and crannies. It gives you the opportunity to enjoy a wide range of associated hobbies—geology, photography, history, botany or bird watching, for example.

Many fitness experts consider walking to be a "best" exercise. Hiking's just a more vigorous form. However, like any other form of physical activity, hiking does require some prudent preparation. The important thing is to begin gradually. Some experts recommend training by walking at least a half hour a day for several weeks before trying a hike.

Once you decide to go out on the trail, you should plan your route in advance and make sure to tell someone when you should be back. Day hikes should begin early in the morning and end well before twilight.

Proper, high-quality equipment becomes more important as the hiker becomes more deeply involved in the activity and tackles longer trails and more arduous terrain. But there is a variety of things a day hiker will probably want to make his journey more pleasurable. The Appalachian Mountain Club offers this list of equipment: a comfortable knapsack; sturdy, broken-in, waterproof boots; a canteen; a knife; insect repellent; a flashlight with extra batteries and bulb; waterproof matches; first aid materials; a guidebook; a map; a compass and food. Clothing should be determined by weather conditions.

Of course, it is not necessary to head for the hills. Hiking can be rewarding in an urban setting. Even in your own hometown, you'll see things on a walk that you didn't notice as you zoomed by in your car.

Hiking is good for your body, it's good for your mind, it's educational and it can be exciting. You can get started on this enjoyable form of recreation simply by stepping out your front door.

An endless selection of scenic beauties are yours to discover when you make hiking a part of your fitness lifestyle. Whether it's a day hike through the country (or even the city!) or a rugged back-to-nature trek through the wilderness, hiking is bound to bolster your fitness quotient—both physically and mentally.

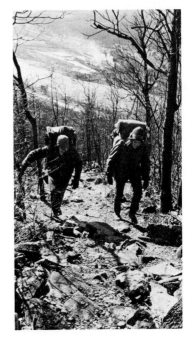

Food for the Trail

You can choose from an amazing array of freeze-dried, dehydrated or super-compressed foods for a day or weekend on the trail. But the best foods may well be those you tailor-make yourself. For a snack, a mixture of nuts and dried fruit does the job well. Complex carbohydrates, like vegetables and whole grains, are good meal choices.

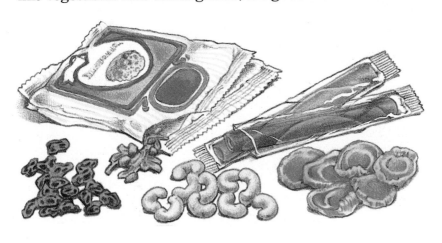

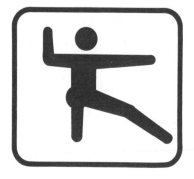

The Martial Arts

You say the stick-and-ball games and all those other traditional forms of recreational exercise are not for you? Perhaps you should turn toward the East and check out the mysterious world of the Oriental arts.

It's hard to categorize the Oriental arts with those strange-sounding names—names like karate, kung fu, judo, jujitsu, aikido, T'ai Chi Ch'uan. Some think of them as sports, some as disciplines, some as arts—and some almost as if they were religions.

In any case, they are very demanding and require as much (or more) mental discipline as they do physical fitness. But the rewards are big, too. Competent practitioners repeatedly exclaim that their entire lives are enhanced by their immersion in the Oriental arts.

In the Oriental arts, you will find many variations on the same theme, depending on the country of origin, and each has its own technique. In fact, styles and systems applied to the martial arts can change from person to person. Describing all the art forms is beyond the scope of this book, but perhaps a few thumbnail sketches will help you get the idea.

T'ai Chi Chu'an. This age-old practice involves a series of 108 linked movements—gliding, twisting, pivoting, gesturing—that blend from one into the next. Slow and graceful, the movements seldom even produce perspiration. Yet they promote relaxation and flexibility, enhanced circula-

The "Supreme Ultimate" Exercise

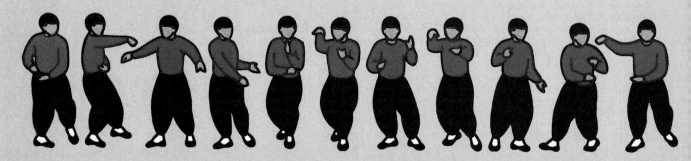

A journey of a thousand miles begins with a single step. So, too, does a voyage into the depths of an age-old method of exercise begin with one gentle turn of the body, one solitary flourish of an arm. And by the end of that voyage—during which the room is never left, no equipment is ever used and perspiration is rarely produced—a person will have completed the performance of a well-engineered workout that loosened, strengthened and even aerobically conditioned. All at once, in simplicity . . . and in silence.

Since the so-called wild times of prehistory, the Chinese people have practiced this quiet ritual. Today, millions of them greet the morning—in parks, on street corners, in their backyards—by slowly gliding and twisting, pivoting and delicately gesturing, to prepare their minds and bodies for the day ahead. This activity sharpens them into alert individuals ready for the workday world.

They don't call it T'ai Chi Chu'an—the "Supreme Ultimate"—for nothing.

T'ai Chi is not a dance, as some writers once suggested. Nor can it be construed to be shadow boxing. It is a series of 108 linked movements, each movement blending into the next, so that the entire half-hour (more or less) routine is one long, unified pattern.

In terms of pure, down-to-earth physical exercise, T'ai Chi is deceptive. It looks so slow and easy, and yet a lot is going on. Hands, shoulders, elbows, fists, palms and fingers, abdomen, hips, buttocks, feet, legs, knees, toes, sides of feet and soles—even the eyes—all are brought into play.

"With the technique of T'ai Chi Chu'an, true energy can be controlled, strength balanced and vitality increased by using the body in such a way so as not to strain the muscles, not to overactivate the heart, not to exert oneself excessively," says

tion and strength; they may even offer aerobic fitness.

Karate. This combative self-defense art stresses hand and, in some forms, foot punching to both defend and attack. It incorporates deep-breathing techniques. Karate is one of the most lethal Oriental arts because it can kill.

Kung Fu. This is the Chinese version of hand and foot fighting, but it involves dodging and long stretching to avoid attack. The idea is to avoid getting hit without actually blocking. Although kung fu and karate are similar, most styles of kung fu are more graceful.

Judo. More a sport than an art, judo is similar to wrestling and has some aspects of the self-defense arts. Its popularity declined as karate grew.

Jujitsu. A self-defense art that combines judo and karate, jujitsu involves chopping, blocking, kicking, throwing and grabbing.

The Oriental arts cannot properly be self-learned. They are best enjoyed in groups, under the instruction of a competent practitioner, and in many cases take years to learn. But the common experiences can provide lifetime rewards through new friendships, acquired skills and a better-developed sense of self.

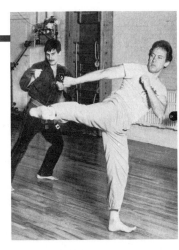

If you're looking for exercise that taxes both the body and the mind, try the martial arts. Karate is only one of the many styles you can enjoy.

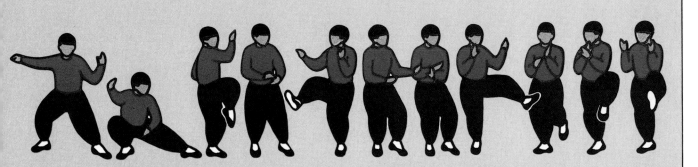

Sophia Delza, T'ai Chi expert and author of *Body and Mind in Harmony.* T'ai Chi develops energy by never allowing one to expend oneself in a gesture of finality.

T'ai Chi is a slow exercise, slow to learn to do well and slow to perform. In fact, T'ai Chi is one of the few things in life that gets slower as you get better at it (and gets better as you get slower at it). A beginner might do the forms, or movements, in under 15 minutes; an expert will take 30 minutes or more to go through the same sequence of flowing postures. The hallmarks of good T'ai Chi are slowness, evenness, clarity, balance and calmness.

But T'ai Chi hasn't stuck around lo these many centuries because it's slow and graceful. Its benefits are numerous. T'ai Chi is perhaps the most mental of physical activities. Through the learning and repetition of its many moves and gestures, T'ai Chi improves memory and learning ability in general.

And yet, it is a mental sharpening that also softens and soothes. You are able to focus to the point of feeling tension and temper disappear. By going so much into yourself, you are taken out of yourself. You never lose yourself—you find contentment and intellectual calm in self-discovery by way of T'ai Chi's repetitive soft movements.

To learn the ways of T'ai Chi and how to float through the forms, head over to the library and read up on it. Then, if you're interested, find yourself a knowledgeable, patient instructor—check the local Y, adult education programs and notices posted at health food stores or Oriental/natural food restaurants.

Do your T'ai Chi at least once a day. Twice is better. Wear loose clothes, or no clothes at all. T'ai Chi alleviates the stresses of the day, while you absorb yourself in the exquisite perpetual motion of shapes you make in space.

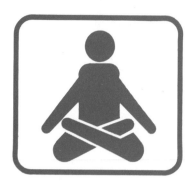

Yoga

Unless you have already looked into it, chances are that you have some misconceptions about yoga. True, this 5,000-year-old practice can be pretty heavy stuff, based as it is on the principle that true health is attained through a proper integration of mind, body and spirit. But you do not have to explore yoga at its deepest levels to find it is a rewarding form of exercise that has been proven to promote both mental and physical fitness. If you're in reasonably good health and need only to tone up, a simple, daily program will do the job.

Yoga is beneficial to all people of all ages, but it is perfect for older people and those not athletically inclined. Further, it is easy, inexpensive, requires no special equipment, is not overly time-consuming and is painless if performed correctly.

A WHOLE-BODY EXPERIENCE

What exactly is yoga? Basically, it involves a series of slow, smooth, fluid stretching motions which, combined with breathing exercises, increase flexibility and promote relaxation. These exercises can be performed alone or in groups and, unlike other forms of exercise, they tone up the entire body while eliminating fatigue.

In fact, relaxation is one of the keystones of yoga exercises. Studies have shown that when you're tense, muscles contract and restrict the flow of blood. This produces swelling, which cuts more circulation. The whole thing's a vicious cycle. But when you are relaxed, fresh blood can flow through the system, providing nourishment and relieving pain-loaded nerve endings. Since yoga

Yoga Stretches

This series of stretching exercises should help you achieve the primary goal of yoga—total relaxation. Begin with your feet slightly spread, bend over at the waist and lower your head toward your

knees as far as possible. Put your arms behind your calves and continue to lower your head toward your feet. Hold the position for 20 seconds or more. Next, sit on the floor with your back straight.

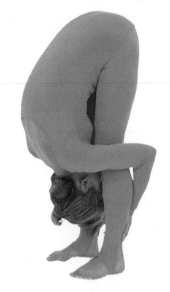

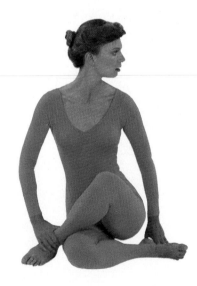

involves those slow stretching movements and regulated breathing, it is ideal for releasing the tension that keeps the muscles bound up. Equally important to the desired effect is a primary rule of yoga: Train, don't strain. It is important to move into each yoga posture slowly and not to push to the point of straining. Improvement comes through careful progress, not by forcing the issue.

Of course, as you get more involved with this ancient science—many consider it an art—you may well want to explore its many other facets. Many claims have been made for yoga—that its various postures are effective treatment for disorders ranging from eyestrain to emphysema, from arthritis to aging—and conventional science is now beginning to find that there is much truth in them. Yoga is being accepted as a serious physical and mental discipline.

Loosen Up—And Relax

You say that life's moving too fast and you feel like a coiled wire? Try relaxing through yoga. This ancient practice puts heavy emphasis on serenity, and even offers a routine to take away tension. The idea is simple. Lie on your back and concentrate on relaxing the various parts of your body, moving from the feet to the head, while at the same time breathing deeply and rhythmically. After proper instruction and some practice, yoga-induced relaxation can improve the quality of your life.

To many thousands of devotees, yoga is a philosophy that offers instruction and insight into every facet of life—the physical, the spiritual and the mental.

Whatever your personal goals—elimination of stress, relaxation, muscle toning, a philosophy of life—you will find that the gentle activities of yoga can offer the rewards you are looking for.

Bend your right knee and bring your left foot over your right knee. Grasp your left ankle with your right hand and turn your head and torso to the left so that you are looking over your left shoulder. Then sit on the floor with your feet together, bend forward at the hips and lower your head to your legs. Grasp your feet with your hands and rest your elbows on the floor. Hold for 20 seconds.

Lie on your back and bring both legs over your head until your toes touch the floor behind your head. Support your upper back with your hands. Hold for 10 to 15 seconds. Increase time slowly to 1 to 2 minutes with further practice.

Lie on your stomach with your legs slightly spread and your hands at shoulder level. Push up with your arms until they are fully extended and stretch your head back as far as possible. Hold for 10 to 20 seconds.

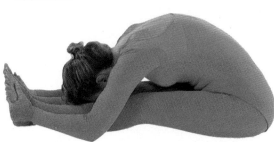

7

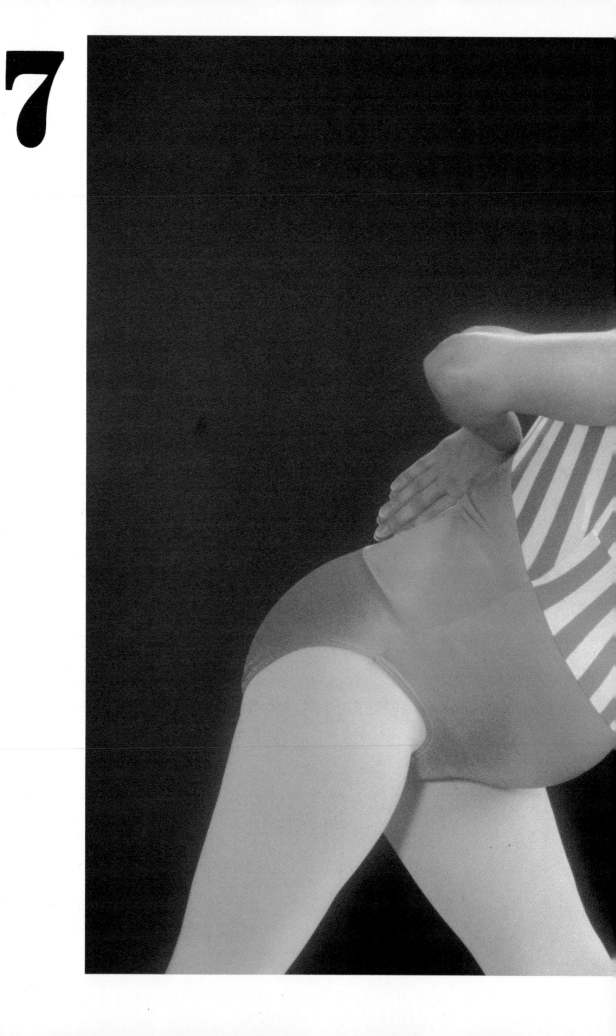

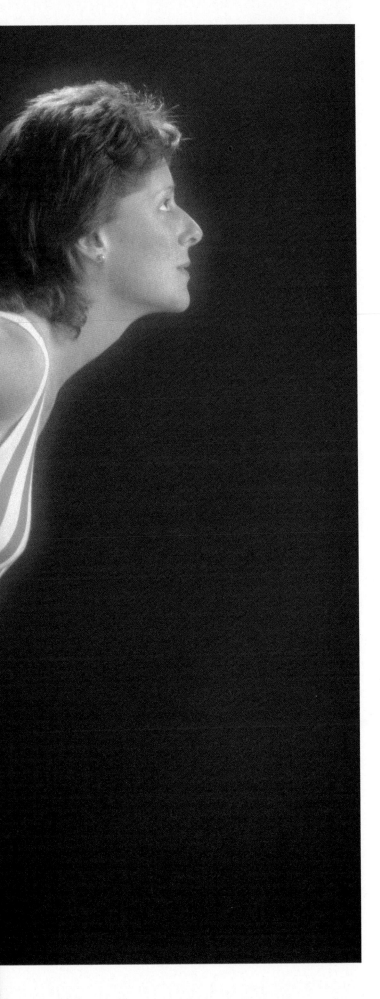

Exercise for Special Conditions

The times when you think exercise must come to a halt just may be the times you need it the most.

In the 1952 Olympics, a pregnant woman won a bronze medal. That's a far cry from Victorian days, when women spent almost their entire pregnancies confined to bed! Now doctors believe that exercise during pregnancy is not only safe for a healthy mother and baby, but that it can also make for a smoother pregnancy and an easier delivery.

Pregnancy is only one of a number of special conditions that can be either eased or helped by exercise. The "exercise renaissance" has awakened doctors to the restorative powers of physical activity for a whole array of problems—from back pain to coronary bypass surgery. Yet, not all that long ago, the only thing people with chronic conditions had to look forward to were restricted lives.

The most glowing example of the medical profession's about-face view of exercise and healing is the role it's now playing in heart disease. As recently as 1966, the standard course after a heart attack was rest—lots of it. The first few weeks meant total bed rest, followed by three or four more weeks of bed rest and relaxation at home, followed by a few *more* weeks—or even months—of "taking it easy" before resuming a normal life. Exercise? Definitely out of the question. In sharp contrast, doctors often encourage heart attack victims to begin an exercise program as early as three weeks after a "coronary event." Six weeks later, it's not unusual for them to be up to 45 minutes of exercise a day, three times a week. That's a lot more exercise than a lot of perfectly healthy people get! Some heart attack victims have even gone on to run the Boston Marathon.

It just goes to show: Almost *anyone* can exercise.

EXERCISE AND ANGINA

Angina pain is the heart's way of calling out for more oxygen. Coronary arteries that are partially blocked by plaque sometimes don't deliver all the blood the heart needs. When that happens, the heart cries out in pain.

How much pain you feel is not necessarily a measure of how narrow your arteries are. Some people with severely blocked arteries feel no angina pain, while others with only slightly narrowed arteries experience angina at the smallest exertion. As a result, people with angina intuitively shy away from exercise, especially those who find that the simple task of climbing stairs often can trigger chest pain.

Yet, this is another case where a gradual program of exercise can help. An exercised heart beats slower and, therefore, needs less oxygen to handle a climb up those stairs. This lessens the strain on the heart that leads to angina.

A good rule of thumb for exercise and heart health is that you should exercise to 70 or 80 percent of your maximum heart rate. That amounts to the highest rate you can reach without feeling chest pain. (This is explained in more detail in chapter 3.) However, for angina patients, a stress test should determine what that rate is. (The exceptions to all this include people with unstable angina, who may experience long-lasting or severe pain, or pain at rest or during the night.)

As you might expect, certain types of exercises are better for coronary fitness than others. Walking, hiking, bicycling and swimming are ideal. Or opt instead for heart-pumping exercise like tennis, volleyball, dancing or racquetball—activities that emphasize rhythmic movement and use your arms *and* legs.

Cardiologists who prescribe exercise for people with angina tailor the program to each individual's limits, capabilities and preferences for certain activities.

One recommended regimen is this: During the first month or two of exercise, people with angina should follow a pattern of short, 3- to 5-minute periods of exertion broken by intervals of 1 or 2 minutes of rest. That is preceded and followed by 5 minutes of warm-up exercises and 5 minutes of cool-down exercises. People may then graduate to a long-term exercise program—such as group exercise classes—to work out three or four times a week for 20 to 45 minutes each. It's important to pay attention to signs of overexertion, such as fatigue or excessive shortness of breath. It's a signal that you should stop or slow down.

In *Mayo Clinic Proceedings*, Charles C. Kennedy, M.D., and his colleagues described the improvement in eight men who enrolled in a one-year exercise program. The men ranged in age from 44 to 50 and all had mild angina. The men met at a YMCA three times a week for 45-minute sessions tailored to their individual needs. They walked, jogged, stretched and finished off with swimming or a game of volleyball. After 12 months, all eight made progress: Three had considerably less angina pain, and five were *totally pain free.*

Albert A. Kattus, M.D., a cardiologist and coauthor of *The Cardiologists' Guide to Fitness and Health through Exercise*, reported similar results in *Medical World News* while a professor at UCLA: "We had our patients walk anywhere from 2 to 4 miles a day, working toward a goal of 4 miles in an hour's time. We had a number of people who at first couldn't walk more than 200 yards without having to stop in pain, but who are now walking 4 miles in an hour, every day, and don't even experience their angina anymore."

AFTER A HEART ATTACK

People who have had a heart attack are even more reluctant to turn to exercise than those who've had angina. They're afraid of the consequences if they don't "take it easy." But, in fact, taking it easy may only make the situation worse. Lack of exercise is no less a risk factor for a second heart attack than it is for the first. If properly done, exercise can help prevent that dreaded second attack from ever occurring. The National Exercise and Heart Disease Project also reported that people who participated in supervised exercise programs after a heart attack had less chance of a second attack than those who did not.

Right after a heart attack, don't expect to be allowed to do anything more strenuous than walking down the hospital corridor. But these first steps are very important ones. First of all, moving about soon after a heart attack helps prevent blood clots from forming in the legs—one of the most common and potentially serious complications of heart attack, because clots can travel to the heart and cause a second attack. At the University of California at Davis School of Medicine, doctors studied 29 people hospitalized for heart attack. Twenty-one were allowed to either sit or stand by their bed during the first three days, while the other eight had complete bed rest. Blood tests showed that the strictly bedridden people had a far greater tendency to form blood clots than the people who sat up or stood for 30 minutes three times a day.

As the weeks pass, exercise plays an increasingly larger role in recovery. Doctors have found that exercise after recovery from a heart attack lowers blood levels of sugar, triglycerides and substances called catecholamines, all changes which contribute to a healthy heart. And exercise raises the ratio of high-density lipoproteins (HDL) to low-density lipoproteins (LDL), a factor that prevents heart disease. Exercise also lowers blood pressure and reduces fatty tissue. Animal studies suggest that exercise promotes the growth of collateral blood vessels—veins that take over for blocked arteries to nourish the heart with blood and oxygen.

All these benefits have the potential to make people who take up exercise after a heart attack more fit than they've ever been in their lives. In a paper in the journal *Geriatrics*, Peter A. Rechnitzer, M.D., says that exercise enabled formerly sedentary people to perform more tasks with less angina. That, in turn, enabled them to go back to work and to feel more optimistic about the future.

Relief from Arthritis

Water exercise, be it 50 laps or wiggling your toes in the tub, holds the key to relief for many arthritis sufferers. Imagine soothed joints and relaxed muscles moving in a fluid ecstasy of exercise.

In the water your body liberates itself from gravity, actually losing as much weight as the water it displaces. So if you displace 10 gallons of water, your body will be around 83 pounds lighter. Those heavy limbs will feel lighter, making swollen and aching joints easier to move. Water exercises help build muscle strength and flexibility as well as fight off crippling deformities.

While a pool's wonderful for swimming laps or group exercise, your tub will suffice for flexing your hips, hands, ankles, back and wobbly knees. So good is hydrotherapy (water exercise) that the Arthritis Foundation and the YMCA have designed a "Twinges in the Hinges" program for arthritics. One may be offered at your local Y.

Dr. Rechnitzer notes that a moderate program of low-level activities such as walking, swimming, golf and cycling three times a week for 30 to 45 minutes at a time is very beneficial. The people who may be ruled out for such a regimen are those over age 65, people with seriously irregular heartbeats, people with unstable angina, people with poorly functioning left ventricles or people with certain back or bone problems that may be aggravated by exercise.

While exercise can begin soon after a heart attack, true conditioning doesn't begin until six to eight weeks after the attack. And all exercise should be done only under medical supervision. It may take as long as a year or two to work up to maximum ability. But the efforts do pay off.

Studies have shown that people who don't exercise after a heart attack are more than 20 times more likely to have a repeat attack than those who exercise regularly. These statistics are based, in part, on a study of 598 middle-aged men conducted by doctors at the University of Toronto and the Toronto Rehabilitation Center in Ontario. The men spent an average of eight months in an exercise rehabilitation program. Their routine consisted chiefly of long, slow running designed to enable them to run almost 3 miles in 30 minutes (or 36 minutes for men over age 45). Of the original number, 498 completed the program, while 100 slacked off or dropped out altogether. Within three years, 22 percent of the dropouts had a second heart attack, compared with only 4.5 percent of the exercisers. What's more, 12 percent of the dropouts died from the second attack, compared with only 2.2 percent of the exercisers.

As with exercise for other special conditions, getting up the nerve to exercise is the most important effort of all: Sometimes the psychological hurdles are much bigger than the physical limitations.

Running and the Common Cold

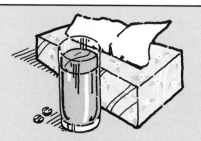

Even runners in tip-top shape get colds, but a mild case needn't curtail anyone's roadwork. Just remember: Be sensible. You need to stop jogging only when certain symptoms strike. A fever, severe cough or earache can mean an upper respiratory tract infection. A severe sore throat may mean you are coming down with strep throat. And a general malaise may be a sign of more serious cold complications.

But with a plain old case of the sniffles or blahs, it may do you good to keep on running. However, take care of yourself by increasing your fluid intake. Use a humidifier to make the air moister so you can breathe easier. A steam bath also might help. Under most conditions these remedies should enable you to run your usual distance.

Finally, don't believe the old wives' tale that colds are caused by damp and cold weather. There's no evidence to prove that this is true. Colds come from viruses—usually passed hand to hand—not from inclement weather.

RELIEF FROM BRONCHITIS AND EMPHYSEMA

Do you get badly out of breath when hurrying, or when walking up the steps? Do you have to stop frequently to catch your breath?

Shortness of breath is the hallmark of chronic bronchitis and emphysema. And it can be very disconcerting: It's telling you that you just can't get around the way you used to. But by giving in to a sedentary life, you may actually be compounding your problem. You see, the less active you become, the "lazier" your lungs get. Your muscles grow weak from disuse, making even walking seem difficult. While exercise may "feel" out of the question, there are doctors who will tell you that exercise is exactly what you need.

Because chronic bronchitis and emphysema tend to get worse with time, it's important to improve lung capacity, build muscle strength and increase physical fitness. The best way to do it is with exercise—gradual, sustained exercise, like walking or easy jogging.

"How can I exercise if I can't even walk out to the mailbox without getting winded?" you gasp. The secret is to begin slowly. As reported in the medical journal *Respiration*, doctors at the University of Toronto and the Toronto Rehabilitation Center set up a program of walking or jogging for 13 people who had either chronic bronchitis or emphysema, or both. All led very sedentary lives and could not exert themselves without getting short of breath. Within a year, 8 of the 13 people got better, with gains in aerobic power. And those who exercised the most improved the most. Their muscles became stronger and they were able to do chores they couldn't tackle before. As a bonus, 6 of the people reported having fewer respiratory infections than usual.

In another study, doctors at the respiratory disease department of the City of Hope National Medical Center in Duarte, California, examined the effect of endurance training on the lung power of seven people with bronchitis and emphysema.

After six weeks, all showed considerable improvement. The advantage of endurance training, the doctors explained, is that it strengthens the breathing muscles. And if the lungs don't have to work as hard, victims won't get winded as quickly.

As little as 12 minutes of walking a day, plus up to 2 minutes of stair climbing, is all that's needed. In a study published in the *British Medical Journal*, doctors worked with 33 people with chronic bronchitis. Improvement was gradual—it took 8 to 12 months before the patients felt the full benefits. But their daily stroll paid off: Eventually, they could walk an average of 23 percent farther— pretty encouraging for people with a disease that usually tends to make them feel worse, not better.

Whether you have bronchitis or emphysema, you'll need some guidance from your doctor before you start to exercise. He or she will want to give you a thorough physical exam and a stress test and check your heart to determine exactly how much exercise is right for you. Walking is the most common type of exercise prescribed, mainly because it's easy and nearly anyone can do it.

A sensible program starts you out at your own level according to your exercise tolerance. In general, there are three starting categories. The easiest starts you out walking for just 2 minutes several times a day. Those who can walk more than 2 minutes but less than 5 minutes should walk daily on a level grade, increasing their walking time by 1 or 2 minutes every ten days. Those who can walk 5 minutes or longer should start their walking program at their own tolerance level. But here you should precede each walk with a few warm-up stretches and light calisthenics. You should also follow your walk with 3 or 4 minutes of the same. This should be done four or five times a week.

When you reach a point where you can exercise for 15 to 20 minutes at a time, pat yourself on the back.

Exercise on the Morning After

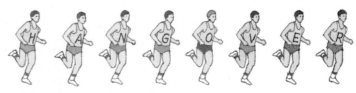

It's hard enough to get out of bed the day after a big night before, much less exercise. You'll be glad to know (and, by the way, so will your boss) that exercise just may save the day. Although there's no scientific research to prove it (and believe us, we looked), there's evidence that a good aerobic workout like jogging can do wonders for a hangover. An informal survey of hard-working, hard-drinking newspaper men (and there *is* research that indicates they know what they're talking about) confirms that the jogging path just may be the best route to take to dispel all the nasty toxins that are playing havoc with your insides and your head.

Whether it's Dom Perignon or Mogen David, drinking more alcohol than your liver can metabolize leaves a number of these toxins hanging around the bloodstream the next day. They must be eliminated before a healthy feeling can be restored. And, the theory goes, heart-pumping exercise pushes this process along.

Exit the hair of the dog.

That's quite a feat for someone with lung disease. But whatever you do, *don't slack off.* To make the walks more challenging, increase your speed. Or find a slight uphill grade for your route.

How far you eventually go is a very individual matter. The important thing is to persevere, no matter how short a distance you go or how slowly you begin. It sometimes takes six months before you see real improvement. Think of yourself as the tortoise in his fabled race with the hare. We all know who won that challenge!

Exercise after Surgery

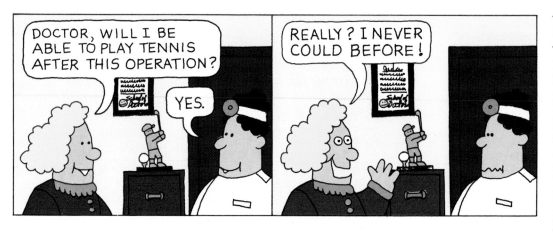

Clearly, exercising after surgery means different things to different people. To seasoned runners and other active people, surgery is an interruption in their normal routine. They're eager to get back in the fitness game. But for people who rarely exercise, anything but complete rest and an occasional shuffle to the bathroom after surgery probably seems unrealistic, especially if they're in pain.

George Sheehan, M.D., the widely published authority on sports medicine, once commented, "There seems to be a consensus that the human body can withstand any sort of trauma in the operating room, but then is unable to do anything more than breathe, eat and go to the bathroom afterward." Yet the truth is that sitting around for weeks watching television is not the healthiest way to convalesce at all. In fact, it can be dangerous.

Exercise after surgery begins soon after you wake up from the anesthesia. It usually starts with a nurse prodding you to roll over, wiggle your toes or even get out of bed and walk. She's doing this for a very good reason—to stimulate the flow of blood in your legs. This important exercise, as little—and as vexing—as it is, prevents blood clots from forming. Blood clots are dangerous because they have the potential to move to the heart and lungs, where they can be fatal. Surgery in the hip and pelvic area is especially apt to invite blood clots. Walking and other leg movement encourage circulation and prevent clots from forming.

BICYCLE IN BED

It's also helpful to bend and straighten your knees, flex your thighs and "bicycle" in bed. According to a report in the *Medical Tribune,* a German doctor has been able to prevent blood clots in many surgical patients by having them pedal a bicyclelike device in bed. In a study of 600 people, those who pedaled the "bed bike" for 5 minutes three times a day had fewer clots than people who didn't. The doctor did point out that they wore compression stockings, which also helped.

Doing exercises in bed also tones thigh muscles, which tend to shrink quickly with disuse. It helps to prevent constipation, other intestinal problems and bedsores.

It's also important not to neglect your lungs after surgery. Your lungs are important because they pump oxygen to your heart and brain. Breathing in slowly and deeply, as if you are filling a container with air, will aid in helping oxygen in the bloodstream. Lung exercise also keeps the air sacs in the lungs from sticking together, thus preventing pneumonia. This is done by drawing your shoulders back and expanding your chest as much as possible.

EXERCISE FOLLOWING A MASTECTOMY

Specific exercises recommended after surgery often have a lot to do with the surgery itself. If you've had a mastectomy, arm and shoulder exercises can prevent the stiffness that generally follows the loss of chest muscle and underarm tissue. Rotating your shoulders, walking your fingers up a wall like a spider, squeezing a rubber ball, crumpling paper into wads and lowering window shades are all important exercises that patients are often encouraged to begin within hours after the anesthesia wears off. Later, when the stitches have been removed, the exercises are made more demanding. The idea is to use the arm, for the more you keep it in motion, the less stiffness there will be from the mastectomy.

Ballet is the perfect way to regenerate arm mobility lost after a mastectomy. It's also a great confidence builder. Perhaps no one knows this better than Jennie Robertson, a dance teacher in Alabama who has had a breast removed. She used her ballet background to rebuild her physical and emotional life after her surgery and she now teaches other women who've undergone breast surgery to do the same. Her ballet exercises emphasize arm movement, but also improve posture and total body movement.

EXERCISE AND BYPASS SURGERY

It's hard for many people to fathom exercise after such an awesome ordeal as coronary bypass surgery. But patients not only *can* exercise afterward, they *should* exercise.

It's important to remember that bypass surgery doesn't cure heart disease. It only relieves the angina pain caused by clogged arteries. There's no guarantee that the new arteries made by the surgeon can't get filled with plaque again. That's why doctors stress attention to exercise after surgery, in addition to avoiding risk factors. Without exercise, there's a good chance the bypass patient may end up with angina pain again—and possibly even a heart attack.

Again, it's not the surgery itself, but the way you treat your body afterward that will determine how you'll feel in the long run. In one study of 349 men who had bypass surgery, activities such as walking or hiking increased by 83 percent over presurgery levels. Men who participated in lighter sports, such as golf and bowling, were 35 percent more active after their operations than before.

Fortunately, it's not too hard to convince heart patients of the importance of exercise. Most people with heart disease actually prefer to be as active as they can. At least this is what doctors at the UCLA Medical Center found out. They conducted a study expressly to follow the progress of people with coronary artery disease—including bypass candidates—who had been following a program of prescribed diet and exercise. They wanted to know if exercise would improve heart health and if the patients would be willing and able to exercise on their own. The answer was yes on both counts. The doctors charted the progress of 64 people for whom regular exercise was prescribed—two walks a day for 30 to 45 minutes each. After five years, 77 percent were still exercising, most of them at least three to six times a week. What's more, doctors calculated that their chances of dying from heart disease were not much higher than those of the general population—highly significant, considering that they'd been categorized as "high risk" at the start of the program.

TRAINING FOR SURGERY

While exercise after bypass surgery is just what the doctor ordered, exercise before surgery may be even better. Noel Nequin, M.D., medical director of a rehabilitation program at the Swedish Covenant Hospital in Chicago, says, "Patients who are conditioned appear to have fewer problems during surgery. They recover faster, and often they tolerate increases in postoperative activity better."

Dr. Nequin has helped to "train" dozens of people for bypass surgery. This "surgery coach" prefers that people exercise for at least six weeks before surgery to lower their heart rate and blood pressure. He adds that the psychological benefits of presurgical conditioning are as valuable as the physical ones.

"Getting back to the exercise program after the operation gives patients a lift," he says. "They feel the surgery was just a temporary interruption."

Fitness and Motherhood

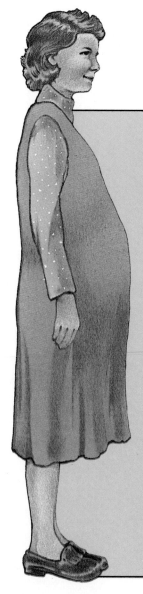

If you've peeked into a health spa or fitness center lately, you've probably noticed an increasing number of pregnant women in the pool, on the track and in the exercise classes. That's because many obstetricians are giving the go-ahead to healthy expectant mothers who are used to exercise to continue an exercise program.

Contrary to outmoded beliefs, studies have shown that in normal, uncomplicated pregnancies, exercise does not endanger the mother or the baby. In fact, studies have shown that the majority of women who exercise during pregnancy are more fit, have easier deliveries and bounce back more easily after delivery than women who do not exercise.

Fear of a miscarriage is probably the most common misconception. Studies also have shown that women who exercise are no more at risk for miscarriage than those who do not. Along the same lines, one report indicated that exercisers are, in fact, less likely to give birth prematurely.

Obstetricians at the University of Illinois College of Medicine interviewed 67 women who'd been running for at least six months before they became pregnant and had continued to run throughout their pregnancies. The women experienced fewer complications and there were less fetal problems than normally expected.

Running during pregnancy has its advantages before delivery, too. It can help relieve or prevent many problems common during pregnancy. In a survey of 195 pregnant runners, many women reported no backache, constipation, fluid retention, varicose veins or excessive weight gain.

But you needn't be a runner to benefit from aerobic exercise and protect your baby at the same time. Other aerobic workouts, such as walking, swimming and biking, are just as safe for the healthy pregnant woman.

Robert C. Cefalo, M.D., Ph.D., director of the division of maternal and fetal medicine at the University of North Carolina School of Medicine, offers some guidelines for exercise.

- Begin each session with a warm-up and end with cool-down exercises.
- Don't get so out of breath that you can't carry on a conversation.
- Don't exercise to exhaustion.
- Don't get overheated.
- Take your pulse every 10 minutes. It should never exceed your aerobic potential—70 percent of 220 minus your age, that is, $0.70 \times (220 - \text{your age})$.
- Taper off gradually during the last three months.
- Stop at once if you have chest pain, dizziness, headache, low backache, uterine contractions, nausea or vaginal bleeding.

After pregnancy, exercise can be an important factor in regaining your prepregnancy figure. It can also relieve the chronic fatigue and low backache suffered by many women

Pregnancy and Posture

Oh, those pregnancy backaches! Poor posture, perhaps? Gail Sforza Brewer, childbirth educator and author, says, "Yes, when you're pregnant, your whole body changes. For physiological reasons your back is more prone to strain. A lot of things happen inside the body, which allow everything to sort of loosen and soften to accommodate necessary stretching during childbirth. And the weight of the enlarged uterus, due to the relaxing of the abdominal muscles, can pull the spine into a curve. Sitting and standing erect will prevent this. It also can improve the circulation." Ms. Brewer suggests using a foam wedge angled at 45 degrees under your back while sleeping as a posture aid. "You will be able to breathe much better and your lower back will be supported," she explains.

During Pregnancy

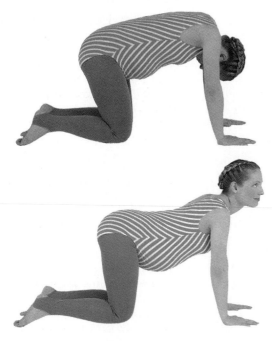

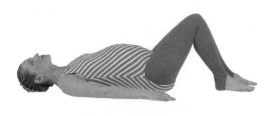

Kneel with your knees directly under your hips and your hands under your shoulders. Arch your back, draw in your pelvis, lower your head and hold for 10 seconds. Slowly lower your stomach and raise your head. Hold for 10 seconds.

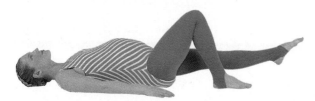

Lie on your back with your knees bent, your feet flat on the floor and your arms at your sides. Straighten your right leg and bring it back. Repeat with the left leg.

After Pregnancy

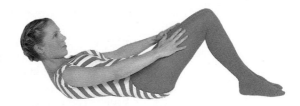

Lie on your back with your knees bent and your feet on the floor. Use your stomach muscles and raise your head and shoulders off the floor.

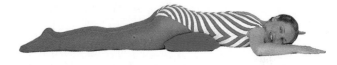

This position helps prevent pressure on your breasts when sleeping. Lie face down on a bed with a pillow under your stomach.

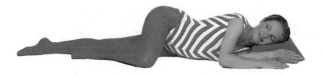

Another sleeping aid. Lie on your side with your upper leg bent and your head on a pillow.

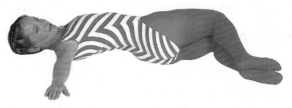

Lie on your back with your knees up and feet on the floor. Slowly roll your knees to one side and then the other.

after childbirth. You may even discover that having a baby boosts your energy level.

A study of women athletes in Germany found that some achieved their best performance after the birth of their first child. The researchers suggested that pregnancy and birth can greatly improve physical efficiency. In other words, healthy women were *meant* to stay active during and after pregnancy.

Exercise for the Aging

Getting older doesn't have to mean putting away the dancing slippers, the running shoes, the tennis sneakers, the hiking boots or the swimming fins. You should get just as much use out of them—if not more—when you're in your sixties as you did in your twenties.

"Age does not necessarily destroy exercise capacity," says Swedish researcher Per-Olaf Astrand, M.D. He believes it is possible to move one's capacity back 15 to 25 years through vigorous exercise.

While some parts of the body decline in efficiency with age, other parts actually compensate by getting *better* with exercise. For example, while oxygen uptake may diminish with age, heart output can increase with training. Blood volume and heart capacity can also increase if an older person works at it.

Keeping your "machinery in tune" can start with something as simple as a half-hour walk every day. "A good, brisk walk will do the trick for the vast majority of people," says Henry J. Ralston, Ph.D., research physiologist emeritus from the biomechanics laboratory of the University of California, San Francisco, Medical Center.

The important step, the "biggest change," according to William L. Haskell, Ph.D., associate professor of medicine in the division of cardiology, Stanford University School of Medicine, "is to get the people who are doing nothing to do something."

Dr. Haskell mentions brisk walking, running, stair climbing, cycling, heavy gardening work and home repairs, swimming and tennis as other possible ways to "rewind your biological clock" with exercise.

In addition, older people should do daily flexing and stretching exercises to keep the body limber and muscles taut. Here we offer a few designed for the older person.

Having a Ball with Exercise

A medicine ball can be great fun—and good exercise to boot! Although these exercises are designed for 2 people, you can devise your own routines so any number can play. To do the exercise at left, stand back to back with your partner and spread your legs a little more than shoulder width apart. Bend over and pass the ball back and forth between your legs. You can either stand up after each pass or continue to bend over, but be careful not to strain. For the center exercise, stand back to back about 2 feet apart and pass the ball over your head, bending as far back as possible each time. To do the exercise at right, stand back to back and pass the ball to one side and then the other, making a complete circle with each pass.

Not bad at all, right? So, why do they call it medicine?

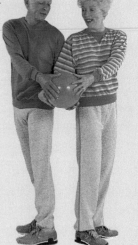

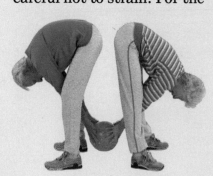

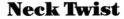

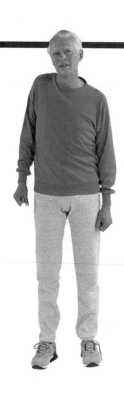

Shrug

Stand with your arms at your sides and alternately shrug one shoulder and then the other. Try to move each shoulder as high as possible.

Neck Twist

Stand with your head up, your back straight and your feet slightly spread. Turn your head as far as possible to one side and then to the other side.

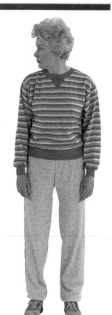

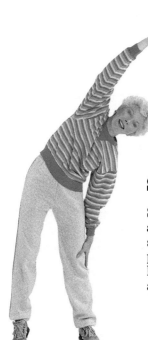

Alternate Toe Touch

Stand with your feet spread wider than shoulder width apart and your hands on your hips. Bend at the waist and reach toward your left foot with your right hand. Repeat by reaching toward your right foot with your left hand.

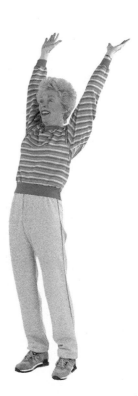

Arms Up

Stand erect with your arms at your sides, then swing them up and over your head as far to the rear as possible.

Side Bend

Stand with your feet spread, left arm at your side and right arm held straight up. Then bend as far as possible to the left and slide your left hand down your side. Straighten up and repeat on the other side.

Exercise on the Road

The exercise craze that captivated Americans at home during the 70s went on the road in the 80s. Jogging enthusiasts pack their running shoes and aerobic dancing devotees tote their tights as they set out on today's highways and skyways for business or pleasure. As a result, the lodging industry has gone physical!

Major hotel chains, including Hyatt Hotels Corporation, Sheraton Hotels and Inns and Mariott Hotels, have included tracks, exercise rooms, health clubs and other fitness facilities in many of their new hotels.

Where existing hotels offer no fitness outlets or have limited facilities, a number of major chains and independents are pumping thousands of dollars into refurbishing projects that include exercise rooms, racquetball and tennis courts, jogging trails and more. And, where new hotels are on the drawing boards or

are breaking ground, generously appointed centers have been provided. Also, more and more hotels today provide jogging maps for nearby areas. To build today without such facilities is like leaving out the lobby or, worse yet, the parking lot.

"Years ago, when people traveled, they lived differently on the road than at home," explains James E. Arnold, director of communications for the American Hotel and Motel Association, which has 8,500 members and 800 allied members. "Now, because travel is easier and people travel more often, they take their lifestyle with them. For many business and pleasure travelers, exercise is an integral part of that lifestyle."

According to Samuel M. Fox III, M.D., director of the preventive cardiology program at Georgetown University Hospital, Americans have discovered something that the ancient Greeks knew centuries ago—the

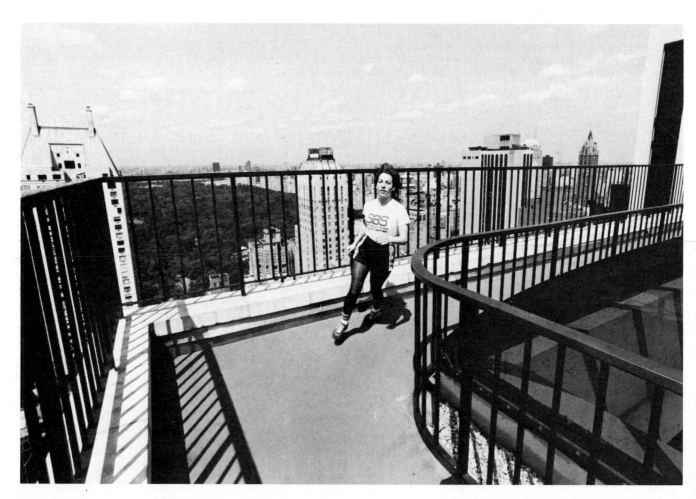

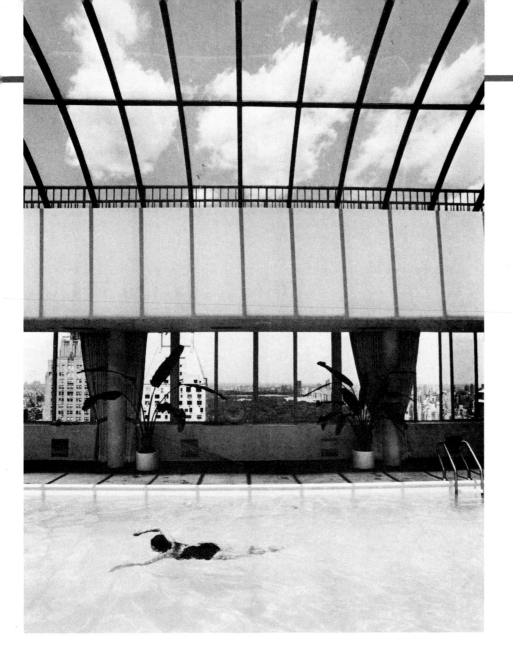

Whether it's a dip in the penthouse pool or a jog around the skytop track, more and more hotels are now encouraging their patrons to bring their fitness programs on the road with them.

importance of physical activity to life.

"Exercise is as important to the head as it is to the body. Positive actions beget positive thought," says Dr. Fox.

Dr. Fox states that the benefits of exercising in transit are more than just keeping up a three-day-a-week workout routine or daily morning jog.

"Very often travelers have difficulties getting to sleep. A good workout a couple of hours before retiring, followed by a warm bath or shower is relaxing," he says. "Exercising dissipates the tension that often arises when traveling. Also, it is tempting when one travels to enjoy a diet that may not be all that prudent. Exercising helps burn off the calories."

After the jogging craze captured Americans by storm in the 70s, hotel managers became increasingly aware that the swimming pool, which had long been the recreational standard for their trade, was losing its popularity. Guests wanted to know about jogging trails, spas and saunas instead. So, hotels began making changes.

Staying in shape makes life on the road easier to take. You have more energy, more stamina and you just generally feel better and perform better. Just like room service and in-room movies, it appears the fitness phenomenon is here to stay. As one hotel official put it, "It's just another service to make guests feel more at home."

Relief for Back Pain

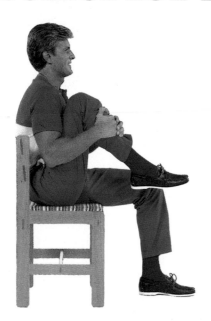

Back pain is one of the most common of all ailments. It's often caused by weak stomach muscles and an inflexible back. That's why exercise is so important. The exercises shown here are designed to strengthen stomach muscles and increase the flexibility of lower back muscles. Make each movement slowly and don't strain. It's not necessary to do each exercise perfectly in order to benefit.

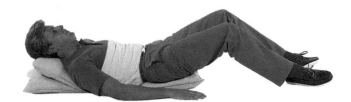

Knee Lift

Sit in a chair with your back straight against the chair back and bring one knee up to your chest as far as possible. Grasp it with your hands and hold for 10 seconds, then relax. Repeat with the other knee.

Breather

Lie on your back with pillows under your head and your buttocks and knees flexed. Inhale, tighten your stomach muscles, exhale and relax.

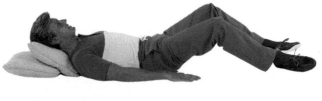

Tightener

Lie on your back with pillows under your head, knees flexed and feet pointing outward. Tighten both stomach and buttocks muscles, hold and relax.

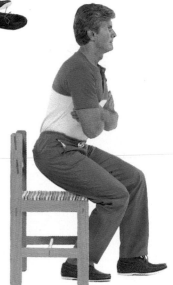

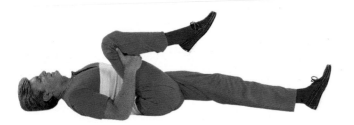

Leg Lift

Lie on your back with your legs straight out. Raise one leg with the knee flexed and grasp it under the knee, pulling it toward your chest. Repeat with the other knee.

Sitter

Sit in a chair and fold your arms across your chest. Tighten your stomach muscles and slowly stand up.

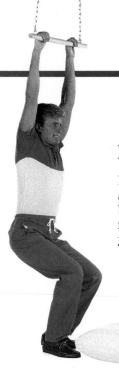

Hang

Hang from an overhead bar with your knees flexed and your feet on the floor until the strain on your back begins to ease. Push your pelvis back, making sure most of your weight is supported by your hands.

Standing Pelvic Tilt

Stand with your back to the wall. Flatten the small of your back against the wall, pulling your pelvis up. Hold for 10 seconds. Relax and repeat.

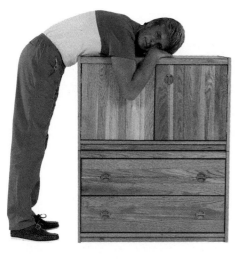

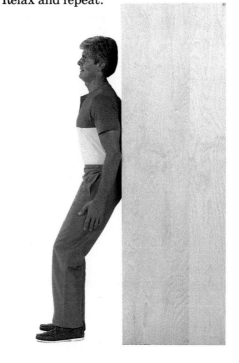

Bend

Use any convenient piece of furniture—one that is about waist high—and bend over it from the waist, lying on the furniture with your upper body. This is intended to take the strain off your back.

Stretch

Lie on your back with your arms extended above your head. Tighten your stomach muscles, bend your elbows and move your hands until they touch the top of your head.

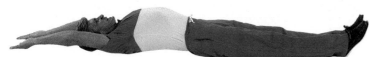

8

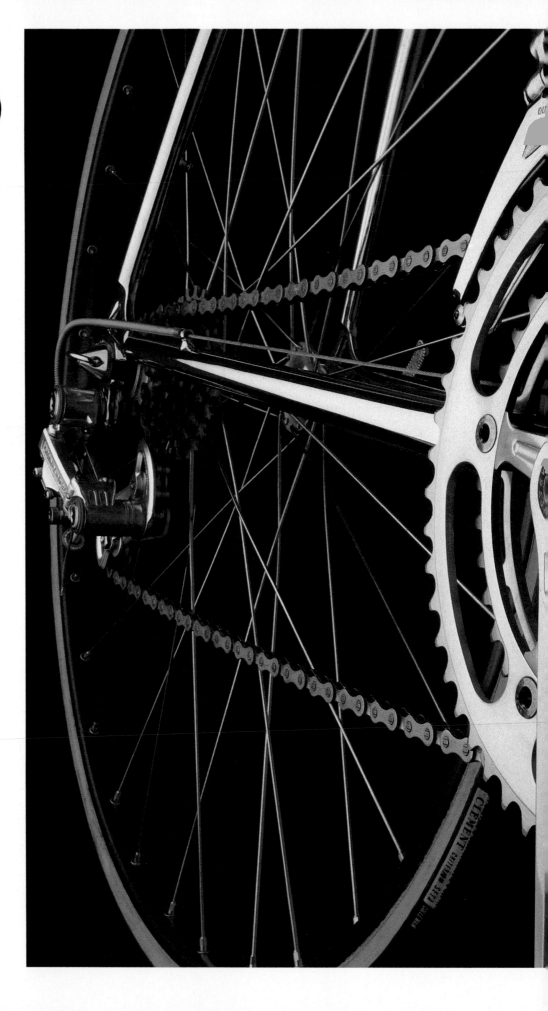

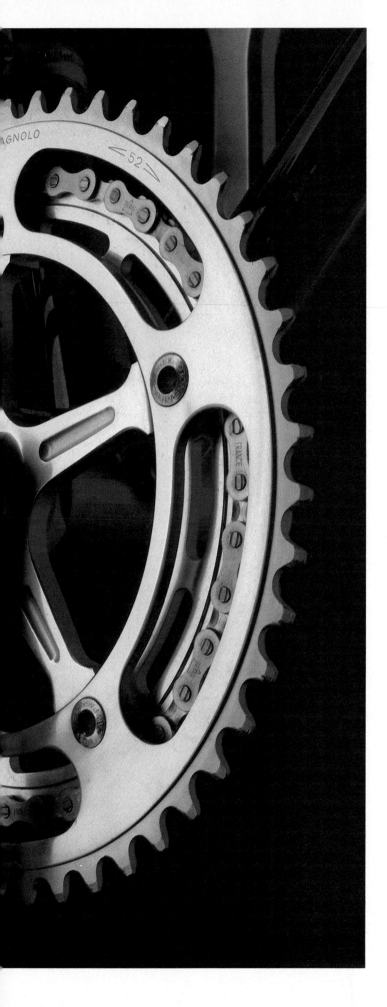

Finance and the Fitness Buff

Are clothes, clubs and equipment luring your fitness dollar? Then learn to spend it wisely.

The "fitness revolution" has not gone unnoticed by the business world. Sporting goods manufacturers, clothing designers, health club operators and even electronics firms have responded to an eager and fast-growing fitness-minded public by flooding the market with an absolutely bewildering array of products and services.

Even a marathon runner would find it hard to keep pace with the rate at which these products hit the market! Electronic pulse monitors that bleep when you exceed your "target heart rate." Joggers' watches that bleep to set your pace. Home gyms. Running shoes, hiking shoes, tennis, basketball and bowling shoes. Lifetime racquetball club memberships. In an odd new twist, there's even clothing meant only to make you *look* as though you work out!

In the pursuit of fashion, it's possible to spend practically everything you earn on athletic outfits and things advertisers claim will make you a fleeter runner, a more intrepid hiker, a fitter tennis player or a more courageous skier.

So, where should you begin? Having a clearly defined, regular fitness program of your own is probably the best way to find out exactly what you need—and don't need. Test a new sport by renting equipment, or borrowing a friend's, before you invest in your own equipment.

To prevent foolhardy spending, you must be able to figure out which purchases will actually deliver enough fitness dividends to justify their cost. In this chapter we will give a glimpse of what's practical and what isn't in the spendthrift world of fitness. Use it as a guide to a life of pleasure well worth the price.

The Best in Dress

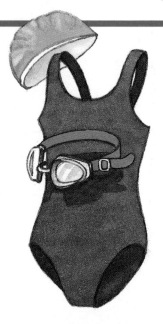

Dressing right for exercise is just as important as dressing for a party or job interview, except that the reason isn't how you look, but how you feel. The proper sport clothes keep you warm (or cool), allow you to move freely and protect you from weather and injury. A sports wardrobe doesn't have to be expensive, but you should buy the best you can afford. Consult a sportswear retailer to get the proper fit.

The only thing that suits *real* swimming is a tank suit. It gives you freedom of movement, and it dries quickly. A cap is the only way to keep hair out of your face. Without goggles, eyes can give out before endurance.

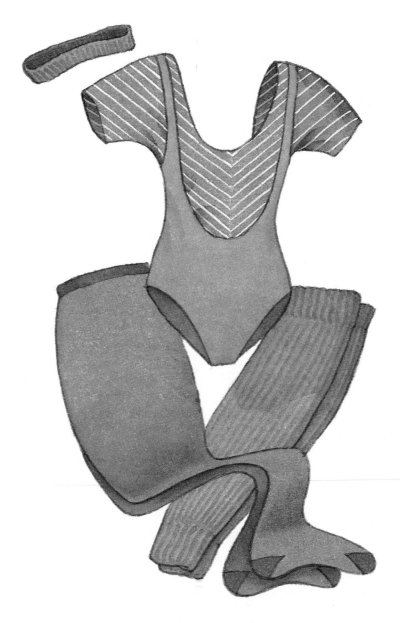

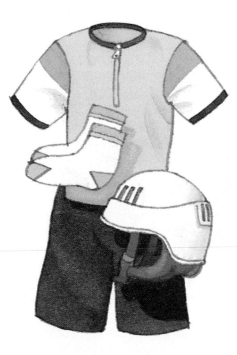

There's much more to tights and leotards than Victoria Principal. Stretchy, clingy, neck-to-toe bodywear streamlines you for vigorous "dancercise" and doesn't bind or ride up the way a T-shirt and cut-offs do. A terry cloth sweatband soaks up perspiration from your brow and scalp. Leg warmers may help prevent muscle cramps by adding an extra layer of warmth.

No one without a great body would want to be caught dead in them, but those skin-hugging shorts and shirts cyclists wear are designed that way for a good reason—they decrease wind resistance and chafing. Cotton socks keep feet cool and blister free. A helmet should go anywhere the cyclist goes.

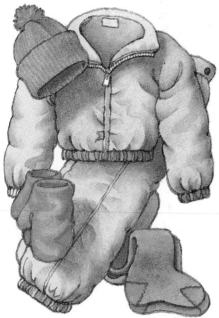

When you dress for hiking you want to be prepared for anything, which is why the layered look is so important. You can just add or subtract a layer or two as the weather moves you. A sleeveless vest gives you warmth, but not bulk. Knickers are great because they're loose and give you plenty of room to move. Socks should be wool, but cotton is fine for the summer. Above all, choose a pack you can handle, with straps that won't bind your armpits.

You want to dress warmly for skiing, but you don't want to be bundled up in a lot of clothes. That's why down-filled outerwear is so important. A cap helps keep in the heat and snug-fitting jacket cuffs keep out the cold. Mittens, by the way, are warmer than gloves.

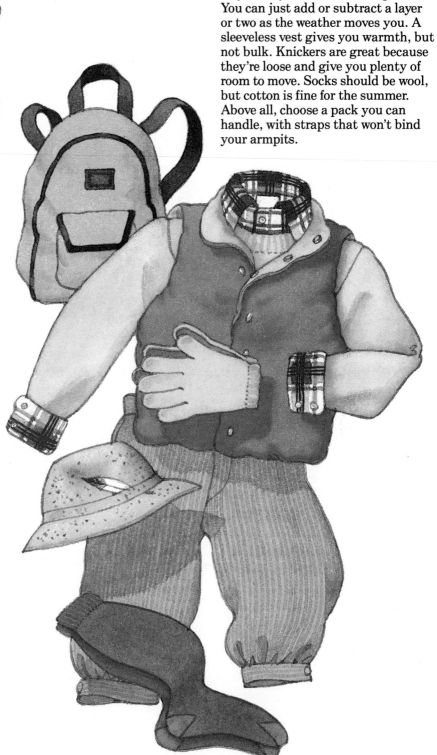

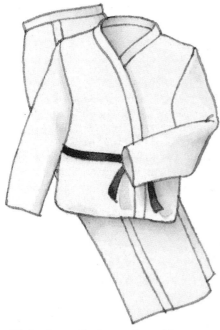

Plain, loose-fitting pajamalike garments are the karate uniform. They're made of sailcloth or duck canvas. Even though they're starched for competition, they leave you free to move and stretch.

The Perfect Sports Shoes

Maybe as a kid you managed with a pair of all-purpose sneakers (probably Keds, right?), but as you've grown in your athletic ability your equipment needs have expanded as well. Today the well-rounded athlete may require—or at least desire—an entire wardrobe of sports shoes.

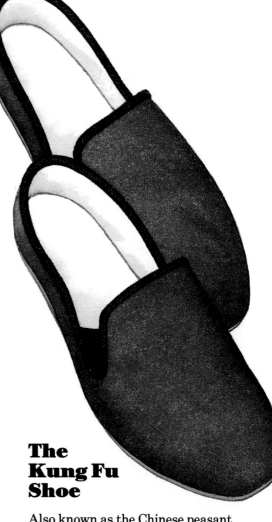

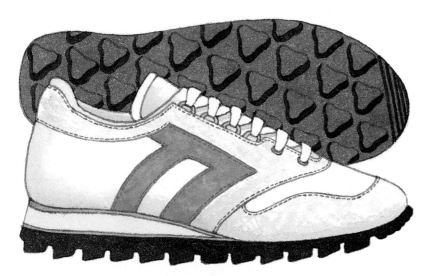

The Best Running Shoe

A good running shoe is easy to find. Simply look for one that's lightweight yet has enough substance to provide good foot support and shock resistance. Uppers made of a fabric such as nylon, reinforced with either suede or leather, fill the bill for weight. Look for a replaceable insole, because this part of the shoe often gives out before the rest. If possible, run in the shoes before you buy them.

The Kung Fu Shoe

Also known as the Chinese peasant shoe, this type of shoe is worn for some martial arts. These shoes provide both protection and flexibility. Made of lightweight canvas, the uppers feature elastic insets that allow the foot full freedom of movement. While the sole and heel are thin, they are textured to ensure firm footing.

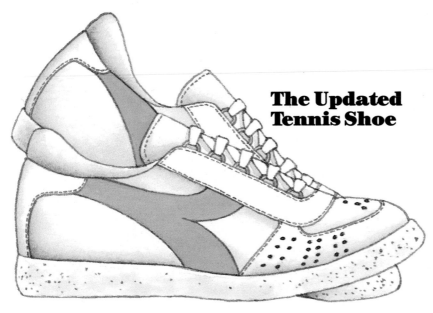

The Updated Tennis Shoe

More than just a Preppie accessory, a good tennis shoe will help you make game, set and match. The intense research focused on running shoes has been applied to tennis. Today's new model is heavier than a running shoe and has an upper that is perforated or made of mesh to increase air flow. Sides are supported with soft leather and the heel features a padded counter. The insole, midsole and outsole also have been improved for support and durability.

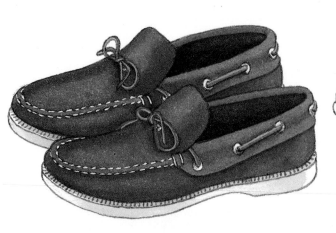

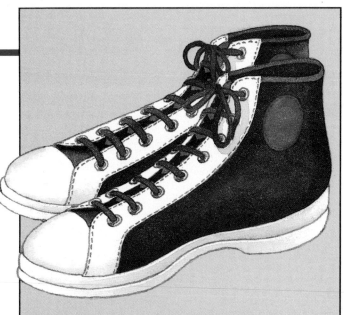

Shoes for Sailors

Decks get wet. They dip and dive. They make for serious falls and injuries unless your footgear holds the boards securely. Look for shoes that feature rubber soles with a traction design. Also watch for thick soles that help to protect your toes as you make your way along cluttered decks. And insist on real leather; as it repeatedly gets wet and dries, it will mold to your foot, making a custom fit. A plus would be to find shoes that have no outer sole stitching. These won't ship water.

In the Beginning . . .

. . . was the first Converse All Star. It made its debut on basketball courts in 1917 and has been a perennial favorite ever since. Although there are many styles, the basic design is still the same as seen on the feet of "Dr. J" and most pros who love the hoop.

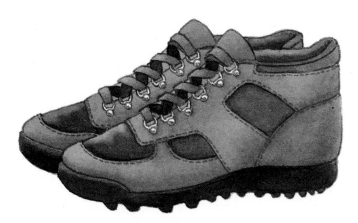

Trail Boots

Protection and traction are the keys to good, comfortable hiking boots. Look for sturdy heel counters, padded collars at the ankles and heavy lug soles. If you are planning to heft a pack, be sure to get boots with high ankles and thick, stiff soles. You'll need the support when you make camp.

Shoes for Cyclists

Unlike any other sports shoe, the cycling shoe isn't made for walking. It's made to fit into toe clips to propel those pedals. There are two types—with cleats and without. Most have a steel shank or other stiffener in the sole to help you pedal better. They also help keep your feet from getting sore over long periods on the road.

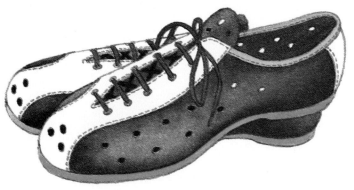

Exercise Aids—Good and Bad

The exercise revolution has spawned hundreds of devices designed to make your workouts better than ever. Gadgets like the ones shown here are often quite imaginative and many are even based on principles of physiology. But buyer, beware! You just may find that what you're spending money on is of little benefit to your body.

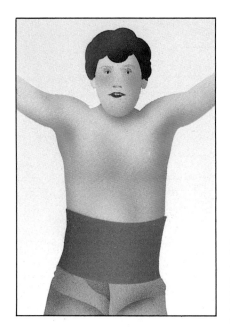

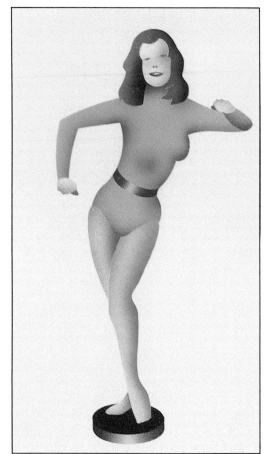

A figure trimmer may be a great device for doing the twist but you'll never be able to call it exercise. For one thing, it's not demanding enough to work the muscles properly. The best way to "twist" the body into shape is with your own power.

A sauna belt may seem to whittle inches from your waistline, but what you're losing is water, not fat. The loss is only momentary. All that weight will come right back as soon as fluids are replenished. Cutting calories and exercising are the only ways to tighten the belt permanently.

A slant board is a convenient and comfortable way to increase resistance and tighten the stomach muscles when doing sit-ups. But you should skip the added expense and the strain it puts on your lower back. You can get the same results by padding the floor and doing sit-ups with your knees bent and your feet flat.

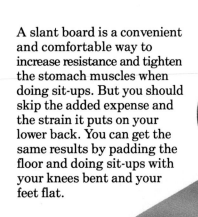

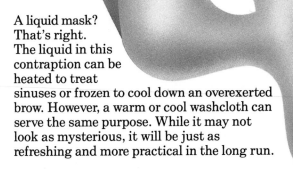

A liquid mask? That's right. The liquid in this contraption can be heated to treat sinuses or frozen to cool down an overexerted brow. However, a warm or cool washcloth can serve the same purpose. While it may not look as mysterious, it will be just as refreshing and more practical in the long run.

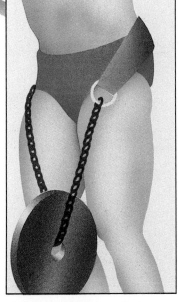

A dipping belt is a device used mostly by those well-conditioned folks who can do 8 or more parallel bar dips and who want to work their muscles overtime. For most of us, however, a workout without the added weight is sufficient to develop upper body strength.

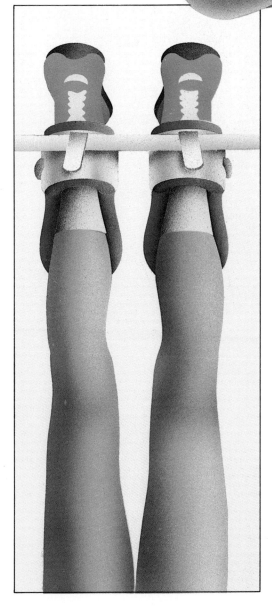

People are going head over heels for gravity boots, which are used for hanging upside down to stretch back muscles and relieve the stress on joints. But researchers at the Chicago College of Osteopathic Medicine say that hanging upside down may be dangerous for some people, namely the elderly, those with glaucoma and those with high blood pressure. The position, they say, raises blood pressure and pulse rate and puts extra pressure on the arteries of the eye, which can be dangerous for glaucoma patients.

High-Tech Fitness Equipment

Just as there are those who cannot drive without a tachometer, cook without a computerized stove or hang a picture without an electric drill, there are folks whose love of exercise quite naturally weds to their love of technology. Their fitness toys go well beyond the basic jump rope to include the most expensive equipment fitness experts can devise and salesmen can sell.

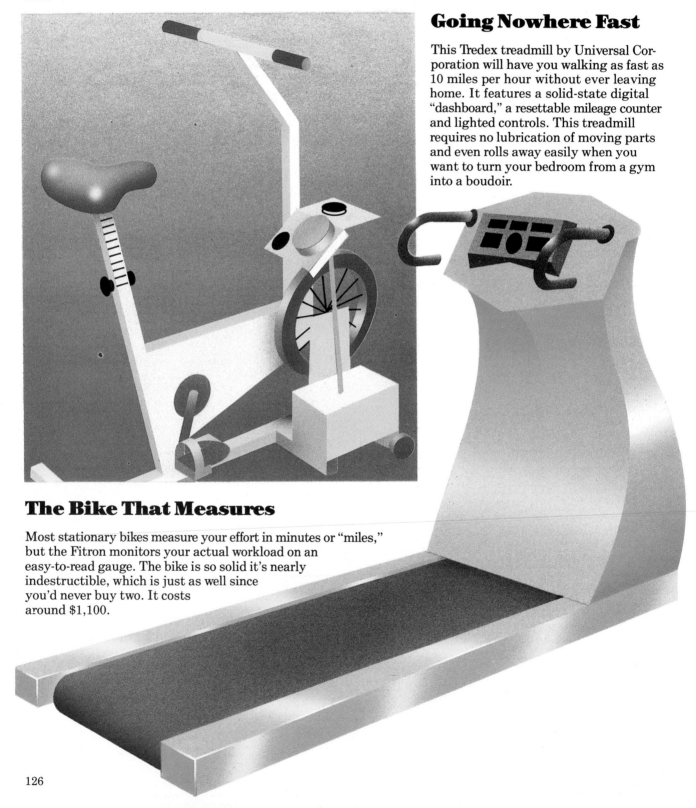

Going Nowhere Fast

This Tredex treadmill by Universal Corporation will have you walking as fast as 10 miles per hour without ever leaving home. It features a solid-state digital "dashboard," a resettable mileage counter and lighted controls. This treadmill requires no lubrication of moving parts and even rolls away easily when you want to turn your bedroom from a gym into a boudoir.

The Bike That Measures

Most stationary bikes measure your effort in minutes or "miles," but the Fitron monitors your actual workload on an easy-to-read gauge. The bike is so solid it's nearly indestructible, which is just as well since you'd never buy two. It costs around $1,100.

The Beat Goes On

One way to know how much exercise is right for you is to measure your pulse rate with a Pulse Rate Monitor. When your finger is inserted into the light transmitter, the machine can read the changes of light in your capillaries as the blood pumps in and out. It then translates this information into average beats per minute.

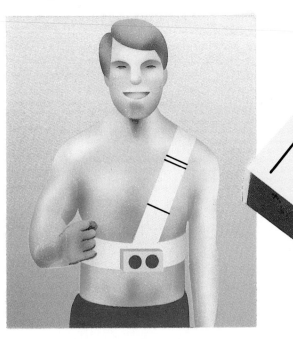

Exersentry Perception

Set the dials for the range in the number of heartbeats per minute you hope to maintain during exercise and this Exersentry belt will alert you if you're slacking off and warn you if you're overexerting.

Fingertip Heart Computer

This 1-ounce microcomputer fits right on your finger and easily goes where you go. It evaluates your heartbeat, showing the results in a liquid crystal display. It also features a stopwatch that tells you how long you've been working at an optimum level.

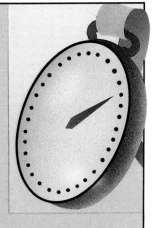

Pedometer: A Walker's Companion

Setting a mileage goal for walking and sticking to it—that's not always so easy. This device—a pedometer—helps you out. Just measure your stride toe to toe, then clip the pocket-size device onto your waist. A small pendulum inside clocks your miles as it ticks off each stride. Pedometers run about $15 and come with a digital or clock face. Just remember that a pedometer will be only as stable and accurate as your stride.

Health Clubs

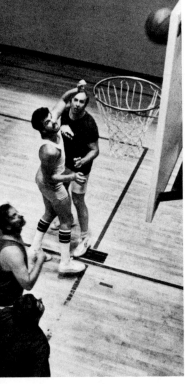

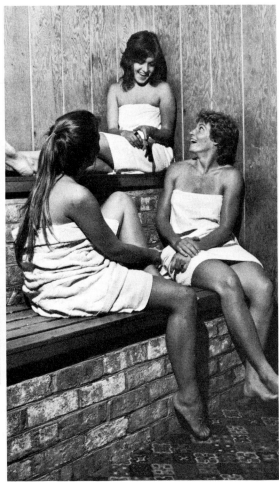

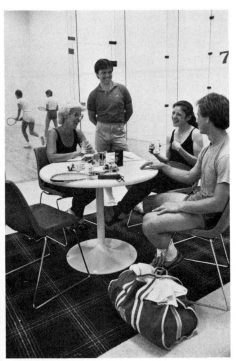

For those who need camaraderie and encouragement to make a fitness program last, it's hard to beat the gym or health club. New friends and healthful success are bound to come your way if you join in activities both on and off the court.

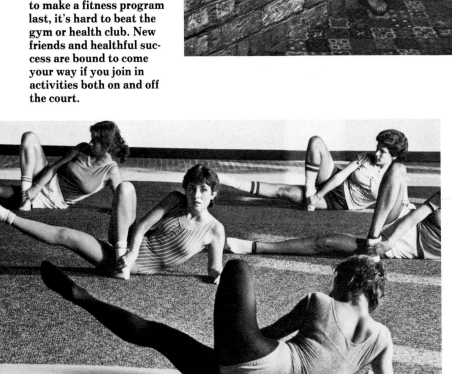

Membership in a health club is not mandatory for people who want to exercise. It's just that some folks prefer exercising in an environment that's a little more elaborate and official than the family den.

But a health club membership *is* an investment, which is why you should join only if you are sure you will really use and enjoy it. Probably the single most important thing to look for is a club that emphasizes cardiovascular fitness—one where you'll find a lot of people running, swimming or riding stationary bikes. That immediately excludes anyplace that claims you can get in shape without effort.

Another major factor is being aware of *how* you like to exercise. If you like to jog, is there an indoor track? If you enjoy swimming, is the pool bigger than a bathtub?

Next, do a little groundwork. See if the place is reputable and has good rapport with its clients. Ask around to find out if there have been a lot of dropouts. Don't just visit the club, but sit down and talk with the manager and interview some of the instructors. Are they cordial? Do they speak authoritatively—and sound like they know what they're talking about?

Ruth Lindsey, Ph.D., professor of physical education at California State University at Long Beach, did a survey of health clubs and found, not surprisingly, that some of them are not very reputable.

Some have instructors with no background in physical education, corrective therapy or physical therapy. It's not unheard of for some places to hire people for their good looks. They're simply given on-the-job training, which sometimes lasts only a few weeks.

Dr. Lindsey found a number of clubs offering exercise programs that are incapable of bringing about *any* changes in weight or fitness. These are usually places that put a lot of emphasis on passive equipment such as roller machines and belt vibrators. Some clubs also have a lot of strange gadgets purported to bestow a variety of health benefits.

"One place had an ultraviolet ray electrical sparking device which was supposed to help you get rid of wrinkles," says Dr. Lindsey. "Another place had other types of ultraviolet equipment, and customers were told it would rid them of stretch marks. That's just not true."

THE FRINGE BENEFITS

Saunas, steam baths and whirlpools are additional health club attractions that may interest you. In a sauna, the temperature is high and the air is relatively dry. A steam room, on the other hand, has the same high temperatures as well as very high humidity. But the sauna may have an advantage.

While many researchers seem to agree that saunas will not help you lose weight, Ward Dean, M.D., a former army flight surgeon in Pensacola, Florida, says it is possible to burn off a few calories. Dr. Dean has done research on the physiological effects of saunas and has found that the body's metabolism increases as it perspires from the sauna's high temperatures. He says you may lose 0.6 calories per gram of water lost in a sauna. So after 10 minutes you conceivably could burn off from 50 to

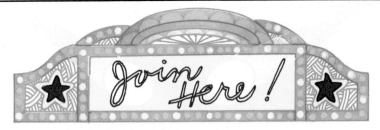

Health-Buyer Beware

To guard against foolish spending, you would do well to keep these pointers in mind when joining a health club.

- Ask if the club has a refund policy in case the club goes out of business. Some states require that health clubs be bonded as insurance to protect the clients' money.
- Forget lifetime membership deals. If the club sinks, so does your money.
- Find out if the club ever has special discount rates for joining or for family memberships. If so, it may pay to wait.
- Never join any club you have not tried out first, or one where the people put pressure on you to join.
- Find out what's included in the base rate. A club that seems like a good "deal" just may end up costing you a bundle if extra costs are added for the facilities you want to use.

100 calories, depending on how quickly you begin to sweat.

While some people say saunas and steam baths make them feel better, they are not for everyone, and their use can be abused. Saunas after a good exercise workout can be dangerous. It may be better to go into a sauna or steam bath *before* you exercise.

A whirlpool bath may consist of portable or self-contained units that direct water forcefully over your body to provide a massaging effect. Whirlpools may help in bringing temporary relief from minor aches and pains due to overexertion, but they are apparently of no real fitness value.

If you do join a health club, you should not expect any quick results when it comes to whittling away the pounds and inches. If you lose a pound a week, you're making good progress. You have to ask yourself what you are going to look like a year from now, rather than two weeks from now.

Corporate Health

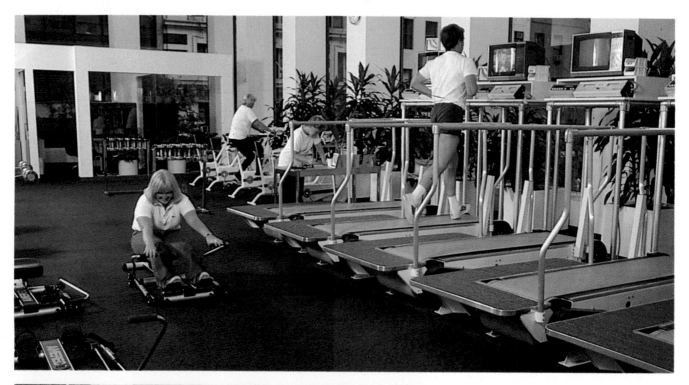

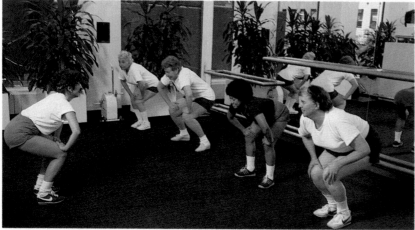

Sneakers and gym shorts in the corporate halls? It was unheard of a decade or so ago, but that was before the corporate halls became decked with gym equipment and fitness leaders. It's the corporate toast to better health.

Not so long ago the vision of the chain-smoking, hard-driving, aggressive-but-inactive Organization Man wasn't so far from the truth. But today, the man or woman in the pinstripes is likely to catch the six o'clock news while pounding out the miles on a treadmill, or carry a spare pair of running shoes and gym shorts tucked in his or her briefcase.

The fitness revolution swept through the boardrooms and factories of American business partly because it swept *everyplace* in America, but mostly because it made good business sense. Most of the

country's multi-billion-dollar annual medical bill is picked up by American business in the form of health insurance for employees and their families. And with the cost of medical care going through the roof, businesses have tried desperately— and, for the most part, unsuccessfully—to reduce the amount of money they hand over to health insurers.

But now, there's a better idea. As former Blue Cross and Blue Shield consultant Robert M. Cunningham puts it: "There's an inescapable logic to the idea that helping employees stay healthy will cost less in the long run than treating them if they get sick." The result? Hundreds of companies across the country now find themselves in the business of protecting and promoting their most valuable resource—the "wellness" of their employees.

Company gyms and jogging tracks, open to workers from all rungs of the corporate ladder, are now increasingly commonplace. Many companies sponsor in-house seminars in smoking cessation, weight loss, stress control and how to do battle against high blood pressure. And such things as computerized, personalized "fitness profiles," with individually tailored exercise programs designed for specific problems, are no longer space age pipe dreams.

The idea seems to have caught on like a brush fire in a drought. Kimberly-Clark, Campbell Soup, General Mills, Lockheed, Control Data, IBM, Xerox and Ford Motor Company are just a few of the giants of American industry that have sponsored in-house programs. Though the payoffs— like decreases in the incidence of chronic, long-term disease— are sometimes very hard to measure precisely, evidence of positive change is beginning to turn up in studies. Fewer work days lost to sickness. Fewer medical claims. Higher productivity. Greater job satisfaction.

One wellness program at Lockheed, the giant aerospace and missile company in Sunnyvale, California, reduced heart attacks among middle-aged male employees by 49 percent over a three-year period, and reduced lost time due to other problems associated with heart disease as well. A Canadian study reported medical cost savings of $84 per individual during one year of a company fitness program. And in another study, participants in Control Data Corporation's StayWell program reported a higher energy level at work, reduced smoking and coffee consumption and an enhanced ability to handle stress.

BECOME A FITNESS ACTIVIST

All of this is well and good for business, and well and good for you—if you happen to work at one of those enlightened companies with the gleaming gyms and the miles of wooded jogging trails. But what if you don't?

In that case you may have to be a bit more ingenious. Judy Kessel's experience at Medtronic, a Minneapolis-based manufacturer of medical devices, shows that making your workplace healthier *is* possible—even without much money or much help.

She offers these tips for getting started:

- First off, it doesn't require lots of money. For instance, you don't

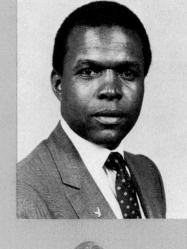

Exercise at Lunch the Gale Sayers Way

How do busy people manage to stay fit? Gale Sayers—ex-Chicago Bear halfback turned businessman—likes to bike 7 or 8 miles in the morning, but he says, "Lunchtime is great for an intense half-hour workout at something like racquetball. You do that 3 or 4 times a week and you'll be fine. After the workout a tall glass of juice with a sandwich or salad at your office is all you'll want." Sayers adds, "That midday exercise and light lunch is perfect for a late riser or the busy night owl."

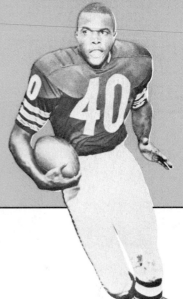

necessarily need a fancy gym to exercise. "You can just push aside tables and chairs in an empty room, or go outside and do it in the parking lot," says Mrs. Kessel.

- It's easier to convince management to go along if the programs are conducted off company time. Eighty-five percent of her classes were held during lunch.

- If you look for them, you'll probably discover that other employees have special talents they'd enjoy sharing. At Medtronic, for instance, an employee volunteered to teach karate and relaxation and meditation classes, "and people loved it," Mrs. Kessel says.

- As a group of employees, you may have more power than you realize. Using Medtronic's potential business as her ace, Mrs. Kessel helped negotiate corporate discounts at the local sports and fitness facilities.

"You've got to be determined, creative and just keep plugging away," she says.

Health Spas

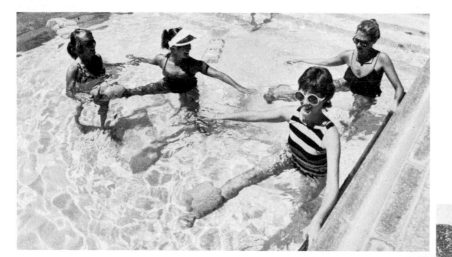

Heavy-duty exercise in the lap of luxury? Incompatible, you say? Well, we can tell you they aren't, if you can find the time—and the means—to hole up in a health spa. These photos will give you just a glimpse of what you may find at one of the country's most exclusive spots, the Golden Door Fitness Resort near San Diego. Daily water exercises, early-morning hikes in the hills and a remarkable herb body wrap—who says you can't pamper yourself back into shape?

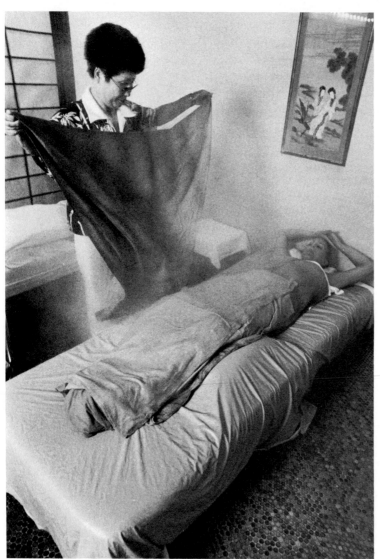

A health spa. It conjures images of rich, overweight women lingering in mineral baths, their faces daubed with mud, while they await the afternoon repast of tea and hummingbird hearts.

It's true that spas have traditionally been places where people—usually rich people—went to get pampered and beautified. But that's changed. The more than 80 spas and "fitness resorts" now open for business throughout North America cater to virtually everyone—fat and lean, rich and not-so-rich, families and singles. Some, however, are open *only* to women, except for "men's weeks" and "couples' weeks," but that, too, has begun to change.

The emphasis has changed as well, from pampering to the pursuit of health and fitness. How zealously the Body Beautiful is pursued varies widely, though. A California spa, The Ashram, near Malibu, has gained the reputation of being "the toughest spa in the country," and rejuvenates its guests with a program that tests the limits of their physical endurance. Elsewhere, aerobics classes and sparkling gyms and pools are simply *there*, to be used as much (or as little) as you wish.

Because fees, facilities and philosophies vary so widely, it's important to find out as much as possible about a spa before you go. Some are famous for their restful, meditative atmosphere but they wouldn't be the place to go if you wanted a week of invigorating exercise, and vice versa. Prices may vary, too, from under $50 to over $300 a day. So study their literature carefully, and try to talk to staffers or people who have been there.

What's a spa really like? A visit to the Spa at Sonoma Mission Inn, an elegant old restored hotel with an attached space age spa, near San Francisco, begins with a meeting with the spa director. At that point, you discuss your personal goals and set up a schedule that will divide your five-day visit into 60-minute segments, so you can pack the most into your stay. Mornings are often devoted to fitness—a warm-up session followed by "slimnastics" or aerobic dance, followed by a hydrotherapy session or a whirlpool bath. After a light, nutritious (and usually very calorie-conscious) lunch, the afternoon is spent in more relaxing pursuits—stress management, massage and stretch relaxation. Evenings are often devoted to lectures about health, fitness or beauty.

At the opposite end of the country, at the New Life Spa Program on Stratton Mountain, Vermont, mornings find guests striding up the maple-shaded back roads in anticipation of an early, hearty breakfast. At New Life, breakfast is followed by gentle yoga stretching to prepare muscles for the rigors of the coming day, then lively group aerobics sessions, working up to the all-important period of sustained exertion. Afternoons are free for tennis, swimming, horseback riding or hikes.

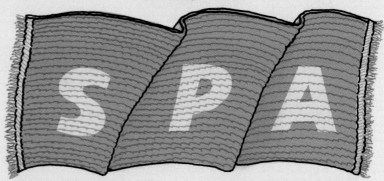

A Day at a SPA

Let's spend a day at the Golden Door Fitness Resort, one of America's most impressive—and expensive—holistic health spas . . .

Our day starts at sunup with a hike through the hills of this idyllic southern California resort. Our bodies limber, we head for an early-bird breakfast of papaya with cottage cheese, wheat germ, grapes and sunflower seeds. So delicious!

Then it's to the Japanese gardens for midmorning exercises, followed by aerobic dancing. Now we're ready for a beauty break—facial, hair conditioning, massage—a true pampering. But relaxation can last only so long, and it's off to the pool for another round of exercise. Before we know it, we're sitting *around* the pool, feasting on a fluffy omelet with asparagus and luscious fruit. Afterward are sauna and full body massage—so luxurious and relaxing—before another healthy workout. An herbal body wrap calms us before dinner. Bedtime can't come too soon, with the realization that we can do all these glorious things again tomorrow!

Late-afternoon yoga and stretching classes are good ways of downshifting from an active day. And when they're followed by a trip to the hot tub or sauna, it's hard to imagine being more relaxed and ready for dinner.

Since so many people go to spas to shed a little weight while they're taking a break from their lives, most spa food goes very light on the calories—sometimes to the point of being Spartan. If you're not accustomed to this, it may take a bit of getting used to. But "the proof is in the pudding," as they say: When your stay at the spa is up, you'll appreciate how good it was by how good you feel!

9

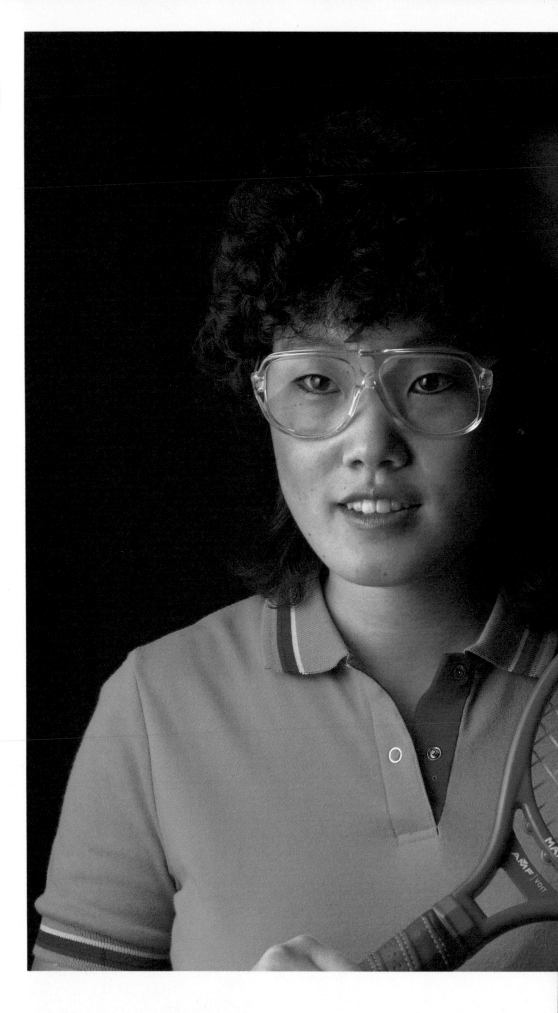

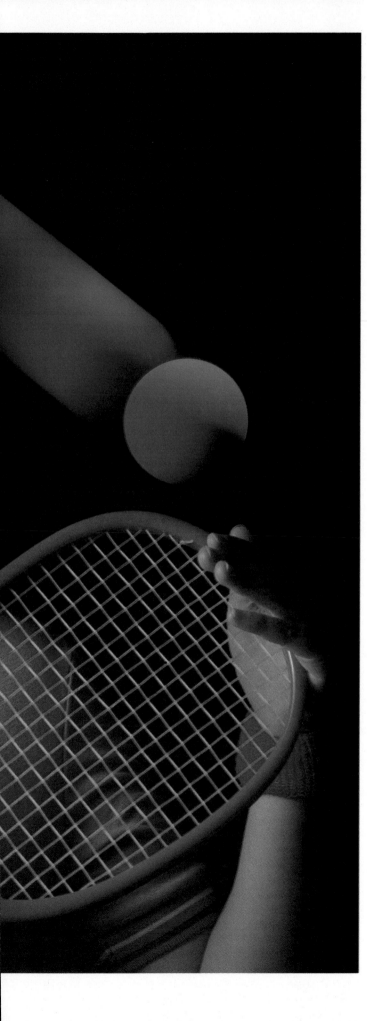

Safe and Sane

Your body talks back to you
when you work it hard.
Listen to it!

Think of exercise as a powerful natural medicine. One that keeps your body functioning at peak efficiency. One that's good for your mind, relieving stress and offering a general sense of well-being. It's hard to envision any other of life's prescriptions that holds the promise of such handsome rewards.

But, like any medicine, exercise must be taken in proper amounts and under the right circumstances. Too little will lead to trouble, but so will too much. Exercise works its miracles best when it is administered in combination with the rest of life's key ingredients. Powerful as it is, it is not the one right that corrects all other wrongs.

Perhaps no one knows this better than Kenneth H. Cooper, M.D., one of the country's leading proponents of cardiovascular exercise. When he first began to jog the nation's conscience into understanding the need for physical fitness more than 15 years ago, he preached a gospel that concentrated exclusively on the value of exercise. He even charted the aerobic value of various forms of physical activity—such as running, cycling, walking, swimming, handball, tennis—so that exercisers could aim for specific fitness goals. His theories not only gained a wide following, they also became rules of exercise by which we still can live today.

But Dr. Cooper's thinking has come a long way in these past 15 years. "As we become more knowledgeable in this field," Dr. Cooper now explains, "we find that exercise is great but not the panacea. I think I made the mistake in the past of saying that exercise can overcome many, if not all, of the deleterious effects of the diet and lifestyle. I believe now that the person who is excessively overweight, smoking two packs of cigarettes a day, but running 5 miles a day, five days a week is in reality doing himself very little good, and in fact may be doing himself a great deal of harm."

So his revised message is one of balance, one which advocates not only exercise, but also proper diet, control of tobacco and alcohol use and stress management. Equally important, he has gotten away from the idea that more is always better when it comes to exercise, and he actually preaches moderation. A strong running advocate, he views five 3-mile runs a week as the maximum proper amount of training. The importance of moderation also is echoed by his colleagues.

Experts and researchers agree that exercise training should be conducted three or four times a week for consistent results. Programs with fewer sessions are believed to have little effect on physical fitness and losing weight. Three sessions weekly have been found to be a realistic goal. Although duration of each session depends a lot on the intensity and type of exercise, most studies have shown 30 to 40 minutes of exercise at training intensity to be optimum.

PLOT YOUR COURSE WITH CARE

Of course, no two people are alike, so the exercise guidelines for you will not necessarily be the right ones for someone else. The goal, then, is to chart a proper course that takes into consideration your ability to engage in strenuous activity.

Medical professionals agree that if you are a healthy, active person 30 to 40 years old who shows no symptoms of major cardiovascular risk factors, all you need before embarking on an exercise program is an evaluation from your regular physician. The obvious first step is a thorough physical examination, but many doctors, particularly those involved in sports medicine, also advocate an extra measure that is not without its element of controversy.

This is the exercise stress test, a procedure by which a patient undertakes progressively increasing levels of activity while the heart is being monitored with an electrocardiograph. Perhaps the most popular apparatus for this test is the motorized treadmill, on which both the pace and the angle of incline are increased as the test progresses.

Controversy over the procedure stems from studies, in particular one reported by the *New England Journal*

The Truth about Doctor's Exams

Do you really need a doctor's exam before beginning an exercise program? If you're in good health and good shape and are under age 30, the answer is no. In fact, Gabe Mirkin, M.D., says that if you are within a sensible weight range and don't have a past history of medical problems, such an exam isn't even worth your money.

"The average doctor doesn't have the necessary equipment to make the exam cost-effective," says Dr. Mirkin. That means you really have to go all out with complete, extensive and expensive testing to detect serious problems. After all, he reasons, "How much can be detected in an office with the body at rest?" Dr. Mirkin feels that anyone with high blood pressure or other serious medical problems should consult a doctor.

But once you've started your program, Jim Peterson, Ph.D., head of the Woman's Sports Foundation Sports Medicine Advisory Board, advises that the best doctor is yourself. "Listen to your body; it'll be rare when the body doesn't declare itself hurting and let you know it."

of Medicine that challenges the test as an accurate diagnostic measure for the detection of heart disease. A study of more than 2,000 heart patients, the journal said, indicated that the stress test adds little to the information a doctor needs to diagnose possible coronary heart disease. Nevertheless, physicians do seem to agree that stress testing has a great value in helping to find proper fitness programs for those over the age of 40.

DON'T TRY TOO HARD

Even with a properly planned and carefully administered exercise program, many people are destined to run into occasional difficulties. Poor training, overtraining, improper diet, extremes in the weather—one or more of these factors can bring on aches and pains that can booby-trap a carefully mapped route to physical fitness.

Far and away the most common cause of sports injuries is overwork. Don't be so intent on your training that you ignore warning signals sent out by your body.

The tendency to overtrain is most common in those who tend to be the most competitive, but overtraining certainly is not limited to the champions and would-be champions. "It is this [competitive] motivation that drives them to ignore pain," says Gabe Mirkin, M.D., a runner and an expert on sports medicine. "I see overtraining not only in great athletes whose livelihood depends on their performances, but also in fitness buffs such as business executives on the squash courts and housewives in a Run for Your Life program."

To be sure, there are super athletes—runners who train 70 to 100 miles a week, ice skaters who spend all day on the ice, swimmers who paddle thousands of meters at a time—who thrive on tremendous amounts of exertion. But they are the exception rather than the rule.

Speaking generally, some of the telltale signs of too much exertion are soreness and stiffness in the muscles, tendons and joints;

FITNESS OVERDONE: *TODAY'S NEW SYNDROME*

The middle-aged marathoner whose obsession with running becomes more important than job, family or even the risk of physical injury may have a lot in common with the teenage girl who diets with such fanatical devotion that she begins starving herself to death. So say researchers from the University of Arizona Health Sciences Center in Tucson, who studied similarities between certain long-distance runners and patients suffering from anorexia nervosa.

A fraction of the 31 million Americans who pursue distance running, the researchers say, develop such an obsession with the sport that "running becomes a consuming goal that preempts all other interests in life . . . Such unreasonable dedication has resulted in permanent disability or even death."

Our culture contributes to the two disorders, the researchers point out: Women are supposed to be slender, men are supposed to be athletic. Though those are healthy goals for most of us, a few seem driven to carry a good thing too far.

depression; loss of interest in training; loss of appetite; fatigue and headaches. When one or more of these symptoms occur, it is time to cut back. In short, it is important to remember that people are limited in their athletic endeavors by the number of workouts they can take in a given time.

To those of you just starting out, of course, the immediate problem is improper training, rather than overtraining. Loosely, that translates into too much enthusiasm. Without proper supervision, we tend to increase the workload too soon, increase the intensity of workouts too quickly, and add new training techniques too vigorously.

Interestingly, all three errors show a disregard for the principles of gradualism and moderation that are now being touted by the experts who see exercise as the cornerstone of a healthy life. Knowing this should help anybody avoid the painful pitfalls along the path to physical fitness.

It may be ideal to exercise 30 or 40 minutes at a time, or to run 3 miles at a crack, but to try that immediately is to practically guarantee failure. James White, Ph.D., director of the human performance and sports laboratory at the University of California at San Diego, offers this advice: "Listen to your body. If you feel the slightest twinge of pain, stop exercising. If you're gasping for breath, slow down. If you can't hum or whistle while you work out, you're probably working out too hard."

TROUBLE COMES IN MANY FORMS

Naturally, the painful pitfalls we mentioned are as varied as the types of physical activity we choose to participate in. Those who enjoy racquet sports, for instance, can easily encounter everything from tennis elbow to eye injuries. Swimmers can run into troubles ranging from shoulder pain to goggle migraine; hikers have to think about pack palsy; joggers can run into a couple of dozen different maladies; walkers have to think about corns, calluses, bunions, blisters and the possibility of being hit by a car. Even the gentle practitioners of yoga have to be on guard against muscle pulls and spinal cord injury. The list goes on and on.

The most common problems are known as wear-and-tear injuries and they generally result from overtraining or from persisting in an activity despite warning pain. While the wear-and-tear injuries sometimes have names associated with specific sports, they actually are common to many forms of endeavor. For example, violinists get tennis elbow and carpenters are susceptible to swimmer's shoulder.

Certain general rules are applicable to the treatment of wear-and-tear injuries, although each specific one responds best to a specific rehabilitative measure. The key word here is RICE — Rest, Ice, Compression, Elevation. According to Dr. Mirkin, a couple of guidelines to remember are that tendinitis responds to

stretching exercises, muscle and ligament injuries require strengthening exercises and joint injuries are treated with range-of-motion exercises.

Sometimes, however, the problems that crop up in exercise programs are unrelated to training methods. You can have structural abnormalities that put added stress on muscles, tendons, bones, joints, fasciae (strong, thick, white fibrous sheets that surround, protect and support almost all the tissue in the body) and ligaments. There also is the possibility of a muscular imbalance that can result when one set of muscles overpowers another set that is supposed to perform the opposite function. Depending on the problem, there often is special equipment or a special exercise regimen that can overcome or minimize the problem.

YOU CAN AVOID INJURIES

Injuries can be very depressing to those dedicated to fitness because the first step in the treatment is to stop whatever is causing the problem. You are likely to be on the sidelines for at least a couple of weeks; longer if your doctor's instructions are not followed. But there is a bright side to the picture. There are certain safeguards you can take to keep trouble from ever happening.

Always remember to warm up before a workout with flexibility exercises, and to cool down afterward with walking and calf-stretching routines. This is because vigorous exercise causes slight muscle injury. As the muscles heal, they shorten, leaving them more likely to suffer a wear-and-tear injury. To avoid trouble, they must be stretched between workouts. Since an effective fitness activity should help to reduce stress and tension, you should try to relax your mind as you are warming up. Also, give your feet a breather at the end of an exercise routine by untying your shoelaces and retying them loosely. If you are just beginning an exercise program — particularly after living a sedentary lifestyle — work into a vigorous routine gradually. This rule also applies if you are restarting an exercise program after

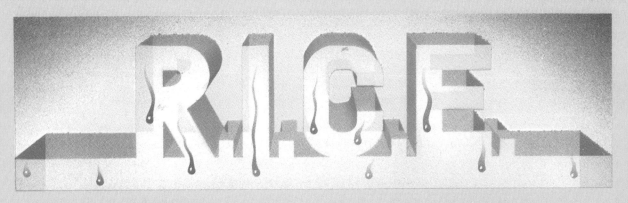

A Simple Icebox Remedy for Sore Muscles

Everybody's had sore muscles at one time or another. Soreness usually means that you've stretched your muscles further than they were prepared to go, but no fibers have been torn. With a severe strain, muscle fibers have actually torn apart.

Sore muscles get better with or without treatment, as do most muscle strains. But you can aid the process dramatically with some simple home remedies summed up by the acronym RICE: Rest, Ice, Compression and Elevation.

Rest means to stop whatever you're doing. Usually, that's automatic because of the severe pain that hits when the injury occurs.

The pain from a muscle strain is only partly due to muscle fiber tears. At least half of what you feel is due to muscle spasms. The muscles surrounding the injured part vigorously contract and hold that position—sometimes for days. This is actually the body's way of protecting itself from further injury: A contracted muscle acts like a built-in splint, immobilizing the damaged part much as a cast immobilizes a broken leg.

As soon as possible after you've strained or pulled a muscle, put *ice* on it. Muscle fiber tears cause some bleeding and swelling. Ice constricts the blood vessels and stops the bleeding, which in turn counters the painful swelling.

Ice also helps numb the pain. But be careful. Ice in direct contact with your skin can cause a cold burn or blister. Put the ice in a plastic bag and then wrap a towel around it. Always be sure there is a cloth between the ice and your skin.

If you don't have any ice cubes available, be innovative. A cold can of orange juice or any frozen food will also do the trick.

Some doctors suggest 10- to 15-minute treatments 3 or 4 times a day. Others recommend using ice packs every 2 hours for 20 minutes. All agree that ice therapy should continue for 24 to 48 hours.

Compression, the third component of RICE, should also be continued for that period, but only if there's swelling. Wrap the injured muscle with an elastic bandage snugly but not so tightly that it impedes circulation.

Elevation gets gravity working for you instead of against you.

Is it a mistake to use heat? The answer is yes and no.

Some doctors believe that the only time heat is an acceptable therapy is when the muscles are simply sore, not strained. If there's any swelling or discoloration, then you've strained the muscle. If there's no swelling, then it's probably only a sore muscle, and applying heat will not only feel good but may also increase flexibility. The important thing is not to use heat therapy too soon. Let your symptoms be the guide. If you've still got a lot of swelling and pain after a couple of days, it's time to see a doctor. You could have a much more serious injury, such as torn ligaments or broken bones.

a lapse of even a week or two. No matter how long you've been an exercise buff, though, remember this one important rule: *Don't* perform the same heavy workout every day. Instead, do what the professionals do. Alternate a hard day with a less strenuous one. It is also important to heed warning signs. A pain in one area—foot, shoulder, elbow, wrist, whatever—is nature's way of telling you to stop the activity immediately. Damage will invariably follow if you ignore the warning.

Finally, make proper preparations for increases in your training activity. This rule applies to *all* sports. For example, you should increase muscle-strengthening and tendon-lengthening exercises before adding mileage to your daily run.

YOU REALLY ARE WHAT YOU EAT

As anybody who has tried to lose weight knows, there is more to it than simply circling the running track or smacking a tennis ball around. Diet is crucial. In fact, Dr. Cooper has come to the belief that it belongs on top of the list. "Your diet is the foundation upon which your total physical and emotional well-being is based," he says. "It's the firm base which enables everything else to reach a state of equilibrium. Without proper eating habits, all the exercise, rest or physical exams in the world won't do you much good in your efforts to develop a healthy body. In fact, without proper nutrition you may not even have the energy to participate in a regular exercise program."

To help you achieve your desired level of physical fitness, the research division at Dr. Cooper's Dallas Aerobics Center has formulated basic principles for putting a healthy balance in your eating habits. They are summarized in Dr. Cooper's book, *The Aerobics Program for Total Well-Being.*

- Make sure that you eat the proper foods in the proper proportions. You will find that your energy level is at its peak if you divide your daily food intake into 50 percent complex carbohydrates, 20 percent protein and 30 percent fats. This is the most important and fundamental of the principles.
- There is another matter of diet division that you should follow to help you lose weight. This is

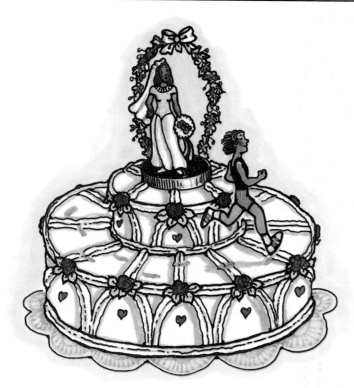

Caution! You May Run Your Marriage into the Ground

Will the pursuit of fitness have you running away from your marriage? A survey of New York City Marathon runners showed that they had a divorce rate 340 percent above the national average. But that's not surprising, says psychiatrist and author Thaddeus Kostrubala, M.D., who believes, "The pursuit of fitness can make profound changes in people's lives and home lives." And it usually happens when one spouse is fit and the other is not. To prevent this from happening, slow down and invite your spouse to participate in a fitness program you *both* will like. In other words, don't keep all those benefits you're getting a secret. Learn to share with someone else.

the 25-50-25 rule. The principle here is to consume 25 percent of your daily caloric intake at breakfast, 50 percent at lunch and 25 percent at supper. The idea is to distribute calories over the course of the day, but to taper off at dinner time. If you don't have to lose weight, you can maintain the proper level by dividing the caloric intake into 25 percent at breakfast, 30 percent at lunch, and 45 percent at supper.

- Do your exercise just before the evening meal. Contrary to what some think, exercising tends to depress the appetite. It's important to remember that, as we said in chapter 1, weight loss resulting from a combination of diet and exercise results primarily in the loss of fat. Diet without exercise results more in the loss of muscle mass.

- Develop a healthy fear of being fat. Researchers are beginning to believe that excess fat, even if it is not a huge amount, may be a more mysterious killer than many believe.

- As important as it is not to consume too many calories, it is equally important not to consume too few—especially if you regularly take part in a strenuous and lengthy aerobic physical activity.

- Know the scientific formula for figuring your ideal weight. Men should figure their height in inches, multiply that figure by

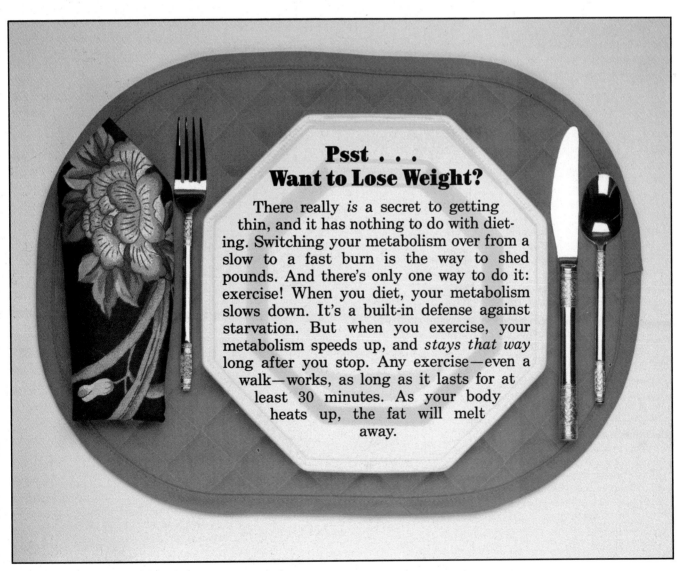

Psst . . . Want to Lose Weight?

There really *is* a secret to getting thin, and it has nothing to do with dieting. Switching your metabolism over from a slow to a fast burn is the way to shed pounds. And there's only one way to do it: exercise! When you diet, your metabolism slows down. It's a built-in defense against starvation. But when you exercise, your metabolism speeds up, and *stays that way* long after you stop. Any exercise—even a walk—works, as long as it lasts for at least 30 minutes. As your body heats up, the fat will melt away.

A pasta party? For one, maybe. Actually, this is a typical meal a long-distance runner might eat in the days before a big race. It's called carbohydrate loading (and it's not without its controversy). The reason athletes eat all the carbos is to stock up on glycogen, the energy they burn up during a race. Without enough stored energy in the muscles and liver, exhaustion sets in. Marathoners call this "hitting the wall." Trainers, however, have found that carbo loading is a way to trick the body into supersaturating the muscles with extra glycogen.

This is how it works: About 6 days before a big race a marathoner will work out at maximum effort for about 3 days. At the same time, he (or she) will load up on protein and fats, but few carbohydrates. This will deplete stored glycogen. For the next few days, training slides off and the diet turns to high carbohydrates like grains, fruits and pastas. Protein and fats are avoided. The theory behind all this is that the body gets so starved for carbohydrates during the first few days of training that the muscles overstock the glycogen that later comes their way.

Carbohydrate loading does have its hazards and drawbacks. For instance, for every gram of extra glycogen the muscles absorb, 3 times as much water collects. As a result, some endurance athletes complain of a feeling of stiffness. Also, all the protein and fat from the few days earlier can cause irritability, fatigue and lightheadedness. And when liver and muscle glycogen stores are used up, hypoglycemia can develop. Further, researchers caution weekend athletes to shun the practice. They say their muscles may not be in the proper condition to take on the rush of glycogen or properly burn off the fat.

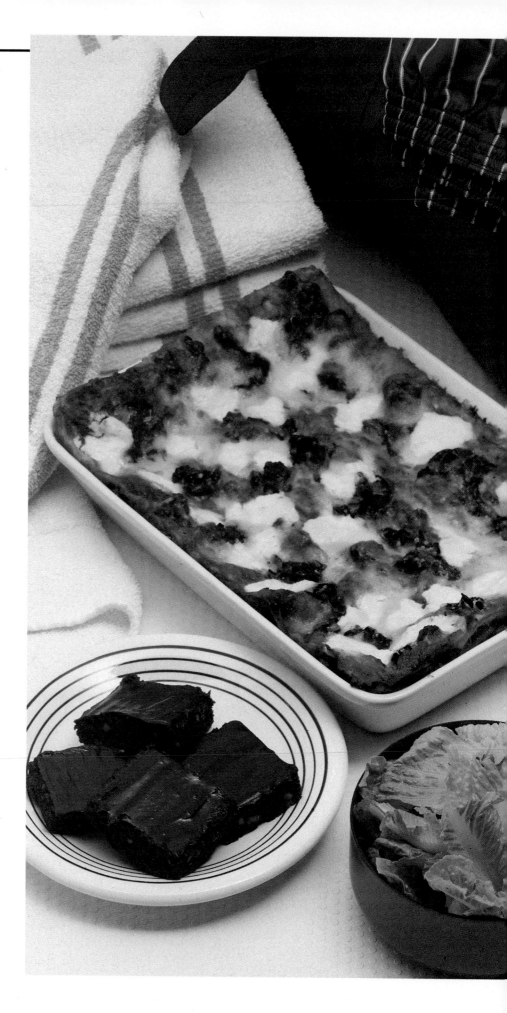

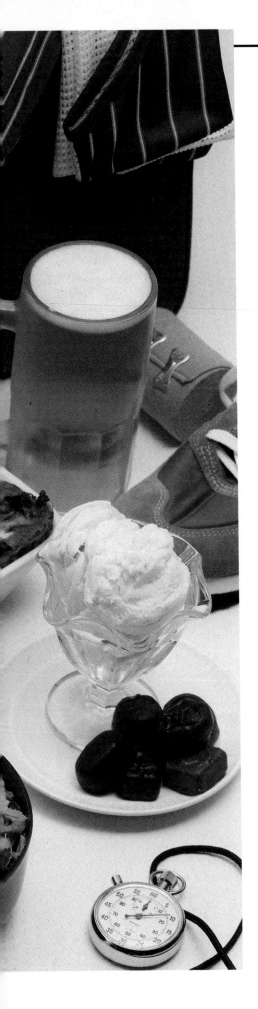

4 and subtract 128. Women should multiply their height by 3.5 and subtract 108. This will give men body fat of about 15 to 19 percent and women body fat of 18 to 22 percent.

- Learn how to figure the number of calories you need each day to maintain your ideal weight. There are variables for the person who wants maximum energy and for the strenuous exerciser, but the way to figure your basic caloric requirement is to multiply your ideal weight by 12 if you are under 40 years of age and by 10 if you are over 40.

- If you are overweight, you should develop a personal eating plan for losing weight. The idea here is to make for yourself a sensible, balanced, lifetime diet instead of constantly rolling back and forth between crash diets and overeating.

THE HOT AND COLD OF IT

Naturally, many of life's most valuable and entertaining forms of exercise — hiking, bicycling, tennis, running, skiing, skating — are accomplished outdoors. For devoted fitness buffs that means coping from time to time with extremes in temperature. You need not refrain from exercise when the mercury in the thermometer edges up toward 100 degrees nor when it plummets toward the zero mark, but special precautions should be taken to avoid serious trouble.

Because the body has the ability to produce substantial amounts of heat, the danger of exercising in cold weather is not as great as exercising when it's hot. Cruising along comfortably in your heated car, you probably have witnessed joggers pumping along in subfreezing weather with little protective clothing. If you looked closely, however, you probably noticed that the joggers were wearing several layers of light clothing, hats to keep in the heat, warm socks and mittens. If they warmed up properly before setting out, these joggers probably were not uncomfortable or in any danger.

Herbert A. deVries, Ph.D., of the University of Southern California, says, "The chief problem in this situation is to prevent sudden changes in temperature (chilling), and athletic dress is extremely important, especially when there are intermittent periods of activity and rest . . . . Athletes must be dressed in attire that (1) keeps them comfortably warm while they are waiting to perform and warming up, and (2) can be removed (in part) after warm-up has been accomplished."

Dr. deVries also notes that the ability to withstand environmental changes varies widely with individuals, but it is a fact that "the round fat person [is] better able to withstand cold."

If you are worried about freezing your lungs with those gulps of icy air, don't. Brian J. Sharkey, Ph.D., exercise physiologist at the University of Montana, gives assurance that "cold air may make your breathing uncomfortable because it is so dry, but there is little danger of damage to the tissue . . . Men have survived temperatures well below 0°F. without damage. The cold air is warmed to above freezing before it reaches the bronchi."

Moving to the other end of the thermometer, you should keep one crucial point in mind. Heat can kill, and it can kill even healthy and athletic people if they do not respect it.

Heat cramps, heat exhaustion and heatstroke are more common than you might think—1,265 heat-related deaths have been reported in the United States in a single summer.

By definition, heat cramps are those painful muscle spasms that sometimes follow strenuous activity. Their exact cause is uncertain, but the fact that such cramps can be prevented or cleared up by intake of electrolytes (magnesium and potassium) and water strongly suggests that a chemical imbalance sets off the spasms.

Heat exhaustion, also known as heat prostration or collapse, can take several forms. "Most typical is a fainting spell in the presence of profuse sweating—usually occurring when persons not acclimated to the heat stand for prolonged periods,"

reports the *Harvard Medical School Health Letter*. "Other symptoms include headache, nausea and tiredness. While persons who faint under any circumstances may temporarily appear to be seriously ill, those with heat collapse soon recover when placed head down and feet up in a cool place. Most important, persons suffering from heat exhaustion continue to sweat, indicating that their temperature control system is still intact."

Of the three maladies, heatstroke is by far the most serious. A catastrophic condition with a mortality rate as high as 70 percent, it raises the body temperature to more than 106°F., causes serious mental confusion and results in nearly complete shutdown of the body's sweating mechanism. The last is probably the most deadly symptom, because without perspiration there can be no evaporation and no resultant cooling of the body surface. In other words, there is little chance of the elevated body temperature coming down.

Why do healthy, fit athletes—including long-distance runners who should know better—get heatstroke? One major reason is basically the same one that is at the root of so many other athletic troubles—lack of moderation. Hot-weather athletes get so caught up in their competitiveness that they forget the dangers of the heat.

The biggest, deadliest heatstroke problem is the lack of fluids. You should drink adequate amounts of fluids before, during and after exercise. This helps to prevent dehydration and overheating by allowing the body to sweat and by maintaining an adequate blood supply to flow to vital organs and to the skin for heat release. It's also helpful if someone squirts you with a hose or pours water right over your body.

So important is the need to replace the bodily fluids lost through exercise that some fitness experts have a simple prescription to protect the exerciser. If you are exercising for less than 40 minutes, just drinking whenever you feel like it and as much as you want should be enough. But for lengthier workouts you can't rely just on your thirst mechanism.

Experts recommend approximately 1 pint about a half hour before prolonged exercise. During exercise, they advise drinking 3 to 7 ounces every 10 to 20 minutes. Water, almost always available, is sufficient to keep the body hydrated in most situations; fruit juice is even better, although it should be diluted with water. An ideal liquid will contain enough minerals to replace lost potassium and magnesium.

One mistaken idea that many people have is that it is necessary to increase salt intake during periods of hot weather because so much is lost through perspiration. This is just plain wrong. But it is important to avoid depletion of potassium and magnesium, two electrolytes vital to efficient operation of the body's cooling system that are also lost through perspiration. This can be accomplished through proper diet. A shopping list for a heat wave might include apples, avocados, bananas, beans, broccoli, carrots, chicken, fruit juices, nuts, oatmeal, oranges, peas, potatoes, raisins, salmon, spinach, tomatoes and tuna fish.

There is one other danger to keep in mind, too, when considering exercising in the heat—sunscreen danger. One study from Texas A & M University's Human Performance Laboratory suggests that creams (those with an alcohol base) that some runners and other athletes slather on to keep from frying themselves might actually only be altering the form of cooking. They bake instead. With sunscreens on, the body heats up faster and stays hot longer, especially in marathons where the body is exposed to the sun for long periods of time. A hard competitor soaked with sunscreen is, therefore, a galloping time bomb.

When it comes to joints, nothing takes a beating like the knees. But, of course, different activities are harder on the knees than others. This chart shows the impact certain movements have on these joints. The weak-kneed would be wise to choose their sport accordingly.

Sports Take Their Toll on the Knees

SPORT	FUNCTIONS OF THE KNEE — Bends	Straightens	Angles from Side to Side	Slides	Rolls	Rotates	Subject to External Force	Total
Ice hockey	4	4	5	5	5	5	5	33
Football	5	5	5	4	4	5	4	32
Basketball	5	5	5	4	4	4	3	30
Skiing	3	3	5	5	5	5	4	30
Soccer	5	5	5	4	4	4	3	30
Wrestling	4	4	4	4	4	4	4	28
Karate	4	4	3	3	2	4	4	24
Baseball	3	3	3	3	4	4	2	22
Running	5	5	3	2	2	2	2	21
Tennis	3	3	3	3	3	3	1	19
Swimming	3	3	3	2	2	2	1	16
Golf	2	2	3	2	2	3	1	15

NOTE:
1 Little or no use
2 Light use
3 Medium use
4 Strong use
5 Very strong use

The Bane of All Athletes: Nine Common Injuries

Biker's Wrist

The constant pressure placed on the wrists as you press against the handlebars can cause weakness in the hands.

Aerobic Armpit

The continuous movement of aerobic exercise causes friction that can result in skin irritation in the underarm area

Jock Itch

Similar to athlete's foot, jock itch is caused by a fungus that settles in the groin and upper inner thigh and causes itching and skin irritation.

Shinsplints

A condition that results from working the leg muscles more than they're used to or running on a hard surface. The pain can be temporarily debilitating.

Runner's Toes

The friction of the front of the toe against the front of the shoe can cause blackening of the toenail. It is unsightly but not necessarily painful.

Swimmer's Ear

A condition common among swimmers who spend a lot of time in the water. Bacteria or fungi in the water invade the middle ear or ear canal and cause soreness and discomfort.

Runner's Nipples

A potential problem for men and women, runner's nipples are caused by friction of the shirt as it rubs against the chest.

Runner's Knees

This sports injury can be a problem to anyone who runs a lot. The pain in, around and underneath the knees is a result of a conflict between your bone structure and your running style. Getting rid of the pain can be as simple as buying a new pair of running shoes or sneakers. A lift under your heel or an orthotic (a customized shoe insert) are other possible solutions.

Athlete's Foot

This common problem among athletes of all kinds is caused by fungi or bacteria that create itching or pain between the toes.

Just about every sport comes with its own set of custom-made aches and pains. The person who wants to spend a life of happy and healthy physical fitness should learn how to identify some of the common problems in order to ward off possible long-term woes.

FOR WOMEN ONLY

You female physical fitness buffs may encounter a special situation if you get involved in a serious training regimen. This is menstrual irregularity or amenorrhea—the temporary absence of menstruation. The bulk of studies on this phenomenon have been made on women distance runners and ballet dancers, but amenorrhea also has been observed in women who participate in other strenuous activities, including weight lifting. Nobody has yet seemed able to pinpoint exactly what causes cessation of menstruation during times of intensive training.

"The most compelling hypothesis," according to a study which included female runners in the 1980

Boston Marathon, "is that intensive running reduces body weight and puts women below a body fat threshold necessary for regular menstruation." But Mona M. Shangold, M.D., a gynecologist and obstetrician, cautions that exercise alone should not be considered the reason for amenorrhea.

"About 20 percent of athletes and 5 percent of other women experience amenorrhea," she says. "In every case it is important to determine the cause. This is because irregular periods or amenorrhea may be caused by serious medical conditions—such as a pituitary gland tumor or underactive thyroid." She also says it could be linked to less serious factors such as emotional stress and dieting.

Joan Ulloyt, M.D., tends to play down the significance of menstrual irregularity among athletes. "As a doctor, mother and marathoner," she says, "I fail to see what all the fuss is about. Whatever the casue of 'running amenorrhea,' there is absolutely no evidence that it is harmful. The absence of periods is not permanent and does not indicate sterility."

As a matter of fact, she warns, "A woman who is having irregular or no periods should never assume she is infertile and depend on this for birth control. I have known several women runners who became pregnant without having a period."

In addition, she hastens to point out that amenorrhea generally occurs only in the young, competitive woman who trains intensely. "The person who is just running for fitness is not going to get this."

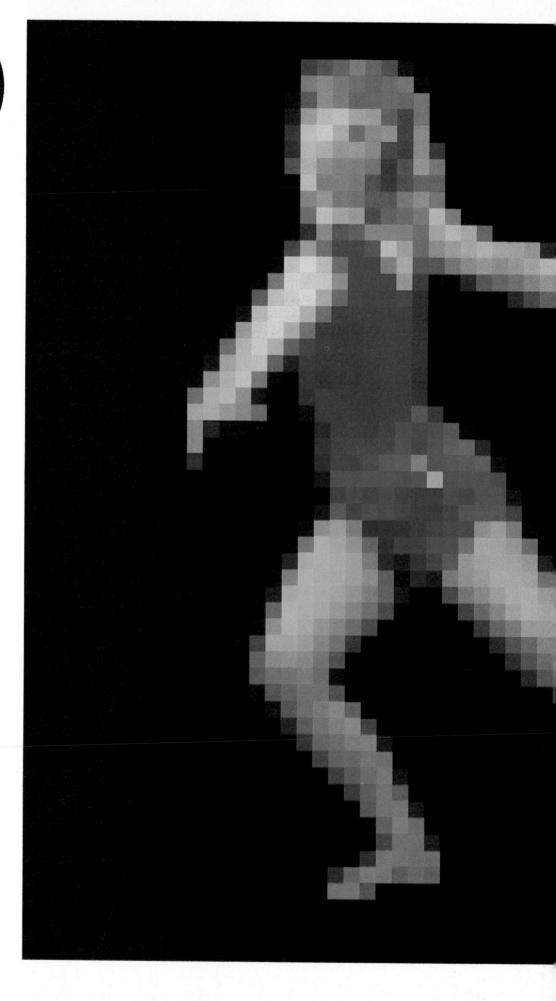

10

Exercise Q and A

Let's set the record straight on some confusing issues about exercise.

When it comes to exercise, it's all too easy to waste time and money. The fitness boom has kicked off an avalanche of new exercise products and promises like we've never seen before.

Sure, some are worthwhile—like a well-cushioned pair of running shoes or a balanced set of weights. But scattered through the maze of exercise equipment is a wide range of great-sounding gimmicks and gimcracks that are long on promise and short on performance. What about plastic sweat suits that are supposed to melt the fat away? Or the vibrating machine that they say will roll it away? Our instincts tell us that it can't be that easy, so why do so many of us keep buying such things?

Well, we don't know the answer to that one, but we do know that there are an awful lot of disillusioned fallen-by-the-wayside exercisers out there who have gone for the easy-way-around-it routine only to find out it just didn't work.

Of course, it's not just exercise aids and fads that thrive on spurious claims. Information about exercise and health also is often distorted, even in idle locker room conversation. Is there really a miracle pill that will change you from a miler to a marathoner? Will muscles turn to fat if you stop excercising?

In this wishful world of easy-does-it exercise, the myths, misunderstandings and misinterpretations are myriad. We want to set you straight on some of the more common misconceptions in the hope that the truth will lead you into a real and rewarding world of physical fitness.

Q. Are there any vitamin or mineral supplements that can improve my athletic performance?

A. Unfortunately, there's no supplement that can shave minutes off your running time or transform you from a fun runner to a marathoner. But scientific studies do show that adequate amounts of *all* nutrients can improve strength and stamina.

And people who exercise regularly may even need extra amounts of certain nutrients, because they put more demands on their bodies than nonexercisers.

For one, the ardent exerciser should make sure his or her diet is high in B vitamins, which are so important in maximizing energy and keeping muscles strong. Daphne A. Roe, M.D., professor of nutrition at Cornell University, Ithaca, New York, found that active people need significantly higher amounts of riboflavin (vitamin B_2) than people who don't exercise regularly. In fact, Dr. Roe feels that exercisers may need double the Recommended Dietary Allowance of 1.2 milligrams daily.

Another important vitamin to the athlete is B_6. Researchers at Old Dominion University in Norfolk, Virginia, found that animals whose diets were supplemented with B_6 did better on muscle stamina tests than animals who didn't receive extra amounts of the nutrient.

Iron also is important in the diet of exercisers—particularly women. Researchers have found that low levels of iron can reduce aerobic capacity and hurt performance. Some 25 percent of women between the ages of 20 and 50 show signs of iron deficiency. And what's more, iron deficiency is common among athletic women.

Vitamin C is another important nutrient to keep in mind. For one thing, C helps fight fatigue. While no direct link has been established between extra vitamin C and improved athletic performance, studies have shown that blood levels of C drop during strenuous exercise. So it only makes sense that athletes get plenty of vitamin C in their diets.

Other important nutrients are: Vitamin E, believed to improve blood oxygenation; calcium, which increases stamina, strengthens bones and delays muscle fatigue; and magnesium and potassium, which can be lost through perspiration.

Q. Is B_{15} the "miracle pill" that some athletes say it is?

A. Forget it. While a lot of money may have been spent on this "vitamin-that-isn't," scientific studies have proven that B_{15}—also called pangamic acid—is worthless. First of all, it isn't even a vitamin—the human body doesn't need it for good health.

B_{15} was dreamed up by the father-and-son team of Ernest and Ernest Krebs. They extracted B_{15} from substances such as seeds and claimed the substance—and its essential ingredient, a chemical compound abbreviated as DMG—could cure everything from eczema to schizophrenia. Its purported powers were exaggerated even more by the Russians, who insisted that the substance enhanced athletic performance by increasing the body's ability to transport oxygen to the muscles.

But rigorous, scientifically controlled studies in this country tell a very different story. In one of the

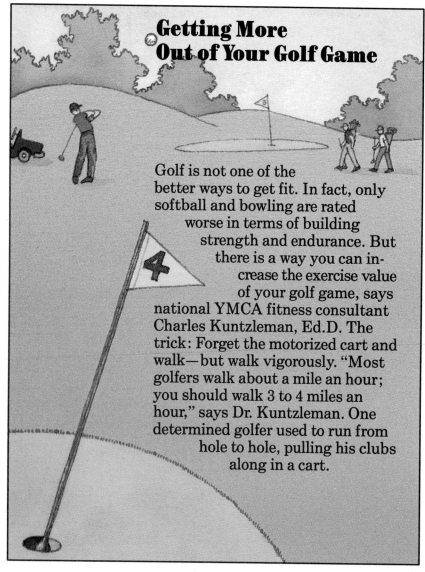

Getting More Out of Your Golf Game

Golf is not one of the better ways to get fit. In fact, only softball and bowling are rated worse in terms of building strength and endurance. But there is a way you can increase the exercise value of your golf game, says national YMCA fitness consultant Charles Kuntzleman, Ed.D. The trick: Forget the motorized cart and walk—but walk vigorously. "Most golfers walk about a mile an hour; you should walk 3 to 4 miles an hour," says Dr. Kuntzleman. One determined golfer used to run from hole to hole, pulling his clubs along in a cart.

many studies debunking B_{15}, researchers at the University of California at Los Angeles concluded that "B_{15} does not result in any metabolic or circulatory advantages for human subjects during short-term submaximal exercise."

But the ineffectiveness of B_{15} may not be its worst sin. Because of its active ingredient, DMG, B_{15} may actually be dangerous. "DMG is toxic when taken in large amounts, and when it combines with nitrate in body fluids such as saliva, it can form a compound called dimethyl-nitrosamine, one of the most potent carcinogens known," says one sports medicine doctor from the University of Washington. "Because of the uncertainty of the B_{15} compound," he continues, "there is no such chemical entity as pangamic acid or vitamin B_{15}. These are trade names for mixtures of whatever the nutrition hustlers want to put together as a pill and call pangamic acid."

Our advice: Stay away from B_{15}.

Q. What about bee pollen? What is it, and does it deserve its reputation among athletes as a "superfood"?

A. While some of the claims about bee pollen are exaggerated, there is evidence that it may improve athletic performance.

Pollen is collected from flowers by worker bees, who carry it back to the hive to feed newborn bees. Because processed bee pollen is high in protein (comparable to beans, peas and lentils) and can contain minerals such as iron, copper, zinc, magnesium and chromium, it is extremely nutritious—for young bees. And it may be nutritious for athletes as well.

In a study done at Pratt Institute in New York, bee pollen was given to 24 runners and gymnasts over a 47-week period. Another group of athletes was given placebos—fake, look-alike pills.

The Pratt athletes were then put through a series of running events and were tested after each event. The results? The athletes taking bee pollen had better recovery power. They regained normal heartbeat, pulse rate, breathing and readiness

for the next event much faster than the athletes who took the placebos. Bee pollen also improved the users' speed performance on the second event.

Q. Can "passive exercise" really help me get fit?

A. It's a nice idea. But unfortunately, passive exercise will get you only minimal results—for maximum expense.

Being advertised as passive exercise is a device called an Electronic Muscle Stimulator (EMS). "It is nothing new," says Joyce Campbell, assistant professor of physical therapy at the University of Southern California. "Electrical stimulation devices have been used for years by physical therapists to treat trauma patients who have lost nerve supply to the muscles, patients recovering from long-term limb immobilization, strokes or spinal injury and to relieve isolated joint pain."

But the role they can play in fitness is another story.

The way an EMS works is simple. You merely lie back and get wired to the machine's electrical currents. Most people report feeling a tingling sensation.

What happens, explains Ms. Campbell, is that electrical stimulation causes the muscles to alternately contract and relax. "There has been no documentation that EMS will help the normal person lose weight, increase stamina or build strength as effectively as voluntary exercise," she says. "And it is no substitute for a regular exercise program, such as swimming or bicycling, in improving aerobic capacity.

"EMS is potentially dangerous and should not be used by those with electronic pacemakers or with cardiac arrhythmia," warns Ms. Campbell. A physically fit body is an active body. Forget EMS.

Q. Should I be drinking special athletic beverages, like Gatorade, for heavy exercise in hot weather?

A. The best thing to drink before, during and after strenuous exercise in the heat is water. It's what the body needs most when perspiring.

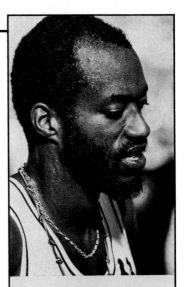

A Case for No Salt

Worried about your salt level after a heavy workout? Well, don't. Salt tablets are necessary only under the most extreme circumstances. Like perspiration losses of 6 pounds or more, which come after long hours— even days—of exercise in the heat. Athletes are more likely to experience cramping from dehydration, or even a potassium deficiency (which a banana or dried apricots can remedy) than a sodium deficiency.

The trouble with the so-called ergogenic (performance-improving) beverages is that they're too high in sugar to be readily absorbed by the body. "When glucose (alias sugar) is made available to an athlete during lengthy exercise, it should be provided in low concentrations," says Edward L. Fox, Ph.D., author of *Sports Physiology*. "The stomach can empty only a limited amount of glucose in a short period of time; if too much glucose is present, the rate of gastric emptying is retarded."

Wolfing down a bottle of Gatorade between sets, in other words, is apt to revitalize you less than drinking a glass of plain water because, to perform in the heat, your body needs water more than it needs sugar. Sugar in the beverage slows the rate at which the water can be absorbed. And that can lead to rapid dehydration.

"A water loss of just 3 percent (that's 6 pints of sweat, if you're a 200-pounder) may significantly diminish exercise performance and provoke heat illness," warns Dr. Fox. For that reason, he recommends "frequent water breaks (that is, every 10 to 15 minutes) to keep the body's water table from approaching that 3 percent deficit."

If you must drink commercially prepared athletic tonics, soft drinks or even fruit juices, the American College of Sports Medicine suggests diluting them with water.

Q. Do muscles turn to fat when you go off an exercise program?

A. This is a common fear among athletes—that an Arnold Schwarzenegger chest will turn into a Sidney Greenstreet stomach if training is cut back. But that's not exactly what happens. You may lose muscle and store fat, but the muscle isn't being "transformed" into fat.

What does happen when you stop training is that your body starts burning muscle for energy, explains Michael Wolf, Ph.D., exercise physiologist and author of *Nautilus Fitness for Women*. And at the same time you're losing muscle, you may be gaining fat because of inactivity and overeating.

"It's extremely easy for the body to store fat, and hard to burn it," Dr. Wolf explains. "It takes 30 minutes of continuous exercise before the body will begin to seriously burn down fat stores. But that's not true of muscle. If you're not exercising, your body will fill its day-to-day energy needs more from muscle than from fat. The muscle isn't turned into anything, it's just used for energy.

"But meanwhile, if you're not exercising much, other things may be happening that encourage the buildup of fat. Often people's appetites don't adjust to their reduced

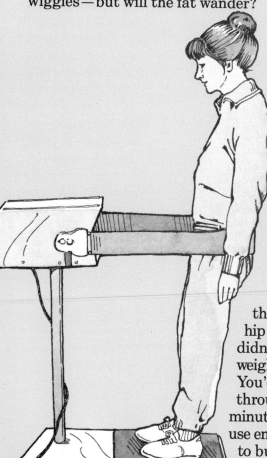

The Vibrating Machine Shake-Up

Is it really possible to shake, rattle or roll away fat? That's the claim made for those vibrating belt machines popular at some fitness centers. The idea is that you lean your tush against a wide belt that's hooked up to a jiggling machine. Your bottom wiggles—but will the fat wander?

No way. An editorial in the *Journal of the American Medical Association* referred to a study on belt vibrators that proved they're ineffective. Not only were they useless in reducing the thigh and hip area, but they didn't help with weight loss, either. You'd have to go through 307 15-minute sessions to use enough calories to burn 1 pound!

level of activity. So they eat more calories than they burn. This happens a lot to college athletes. After they graduate and stop playing, they still eat the same way they did at the training table—and they wind up replacing muscle with fat."

If you have big muscles, are planning to cut back on training and don't want to reckon with a lot of flab, be sure to reduce your intake of calories and try to get some aerobic exercise.

Q. Is it a good idea to eat a candy bar or other sugary food for energy just before exercise or an athletic event?

A. No. Eating sweets just prior to exercise sets you up for a sugar rebound effect. "If you eat a doughnut or drink a soft drink, your blood sugar level will go up, temporarily giving you more energy," says exercise physiologist and national YMCA fitness consultant Charles Kuntzleman, Ed.D. "But the sugar level goes too high. So, the body then releases insulin, a hormone that brings the blood sugar level down. However, the body tends to overcompensate with insulin—your blood sugar will drop so low that you'll actually run *out* of energy."

Q. Does it help, when trying to lose weight, to exercise in a plastic sweat suit?

A. No. In fact, plastic sweat suits can be dangerous, especially if they're used in hot weather.

The appeal of those suits is that they make you sweat—plenty—so you'll experience a rapid weight loss. That's why athletes who have to be below a certain weight—like wrestlers—sometimes use them shortly before their weigh-in.

But as those athletes know, the loss is *all* water, *no* fat, and *very* temporary— the water comes right back from food and drink after exercise.

The vinyl sweat suits also interfere with the body's natural temperature-regulating process. Perspiration comes to the surface of your skin for a reason—to be evaporated and cool you. But wrap yourself in plastic gear and you choke off

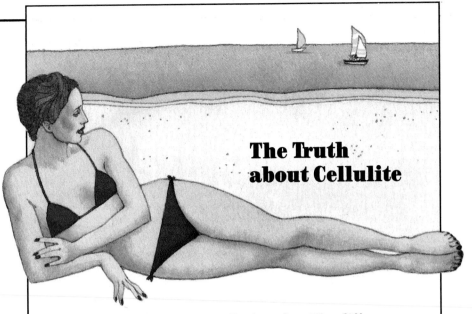

The Truth about Cellulite

What is cellulite? It's really just fat. The difference is that the fat develops in little pockets. Fibrous bands appear between the pockets and the skin, creating a rippled effect—like a balloon pressed against a tennis racket. The way you get rid of cellulite is the way you get rid of any fat—by eating less and getting aerobic exercise. Massage may also help, by encouraging blood flow and breaking up the fibrous bands. Avoiding tight clothing and not crossing your legs also helps.

the air flow needed to do that. The danger of heatstroke is very real.

Q. Can weekend workouts keep me fit?

A. Yes. If you exercise just two consecutive days a week, you can achieve a reasonable level of fitness.

That may sound like health heresy, compared to the "at least three days a week" prescription we've been talking about, but according to exercise experts Arthur Weltman, Ph.D., and Bryant Stamford, Ph.D., it is possible—and practical.

"The idea for weekend exercise came after hearing so often from people that they were just 'too busy' to exercise consistently during the week because of their jobs," says Dr. Stamford. "From our research and the results of others, we concluded that exercising just two days a week can produce very positive results."

But you have to do it right. To get fit on weekends—and avoid the aches and pains normally associated with overly enthusiastic weekend exercise— you should build up your level of exercise slowly.

Swimming and bicycling are ideal weekend exercises because they don't put heavy stress on joints. Dr. Stamford suggests starting with 15 minutes at whatever pace you can handle. Add a few more minutes each weekend until you are swimming or cycling for 1 hour per session.

If jogging is your preferred sport, you should progress more slowly, since jogging places a greater strain on the joints. Dr. Stamford recommends that you start your weekend fitness program with ½ mile of vigorous walking—or mixed walking and jogging—both days for the first two weekends. Within a month or so, build up to a mile a day of mixed walking and jogging. Gradually increase mileage and jogging distance.

In as little as four months, you should be able to jog for 3 miles— and that's the level you should stay at if you exercise only two days a week. "You simply can't do big mileage on weekend-only conditioning," says Dr. Stamford.

How fit will you be with a weekend-only regimen? If you're already fit, you can maintain that level of fitness. If you're not in such good shape, you can become aerobically fit—meaning your body will be using oxygen more efficiently and your heart will be stronger. However, you probably won't lose much weight— studies indicate that at least three days of exercise per week are needed to lose significant amounts of fat.

Q. Can exercise erase the bad effects of smoking?

A. No—and in fact, the opposite may be true. Cigarette smoking may undo one of the key benefits of exercise— reduced risk of heart disease.

Nonsmokers who exercise have a healthy, high level of HDL cholesterol, the "good" cholesterol that wards off heart disease. But a study at the University of Louisville in Kentucky found that people who smoke more than a pack of cigarettes a day and also exercise still have low, unhealthy levels of HDL cholesterol.

The implication in terms of reduced risk of heart attack is that exercise probably won't do much good for someone who continues to smoke heavily.

But that doesn't mean smokers should throw in their sweat towels. Exercise still benefits them in other ways. For example, it relieves stress and keeps body fat down—which is especially important when people are trying to quit smoking. Many former smokers finally broke the cigarette habit by taking up a new and healthier exercise habit.

Q. How long does it really take to get in shape?

A. Probably not as long as you think. Even if you haven't exercised for ten years, don't think you're a lost cause. You can be in really decent shape in just two months.

The Muscle-Bound Myth

You *can* have big muscles and also be limber. "'Muscle-bound' is a myth," says Michael Wolf, Ph.D., exercise physiologist and weight training expert. "There's no necessary correlation between muscle size and flexibility."

Then why has the myth persisted so long? Dr. Wolf explains that in days gone by, muscle-men used "free weights" —like barbells—and often didn't exercise their muscles through a complete range of motion. That made them stiff. But today's more sophisticated weight machines encourage you to bring muscles through their full range. Plus, many body builders do flexibility exercises. The result? Many of the largest body builders can tie their bodies in knots.

Researchers at Arizona State University and the University of Western Ontario tested formerly active men between the ages of 30 and 39. These people hadn't lifted a weight or run a mile in ten years or more. But once they put their running shoes back on and exercised three times a week for eight weeks, their endurance came right back up to high levels of fitness. A never-active group also enjoyed healthy increases in fitness in eight weeks.

Another study, with younger subjects, showed even faster results. John Pearn, M.D., an Australian physician, put 50 untrained male college students through 20 minutes of exercise a day—and in only 14 days, "all the subjects became fit . . . with objective improvement in both absolute strength and pulse recovery time." Dr. Pearn's program consisted of three sets of ten exercises, including chin-ups, weight lifting, and step climbing, which the men went through as quickly as they comfortably could, usually 10 minutes, twice a day. Total exercise time over the two-week period came to only about 6 hours.

Of course, the older and more out of shape you are, the longer it will—and should—take to get fit, since you don't want to push yourself too hard. But it is nice to know that the road to fitness really isn't all that long.

Q. Are steam baths and saunas good for the body?

A. Exposure to heat in the form of either a steam bath or a sauna amounts essentially to a workout for your body's thermal regulation system. Writing in the *Journal of the American Medical Association*, David I. Abramson, M.D., reports that "in

The Natural High

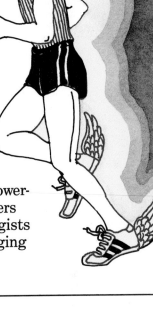

Many a runner has experienced it. "Runner's high" is that breezy elation that begins after several minutes of exercise and may last until well after a session has ended.

There are plenty of theories about possible biological origins of this joy. One is that it's brought on by an array of chemicals—including endorphins, morphinelike substances—that the body secretes during exercise.

Whatever the cause, it's a powerful phenomenon that keeps runners trotting back for more. Psychologists are even finding that regular jogging can cure depression.

normal subjects, there are increases in cardiac output, pulse rate and central venous pressure, and decreases in circulation time, systolic pressure and peripheral resistance." What that means is your heart pumps more blood to your skin, for cooling purposes, and less to your internal organs. "There is also a considerable depletion of salt from the body through perspiration," Dr. Abramson notes, "and in hypertensive patients, a noteworthy fall in both systolic and diastolic blood pressure occurs."

However, Dr. Abramson feels that steam baths and saunas should be used by the sound of heart only. If you have any serious organic disability, such as generalized arteriosclerosis, chronic pulmonary disorders, cardiac difficulties or hyperthyroidism, you should stay away from them.

11

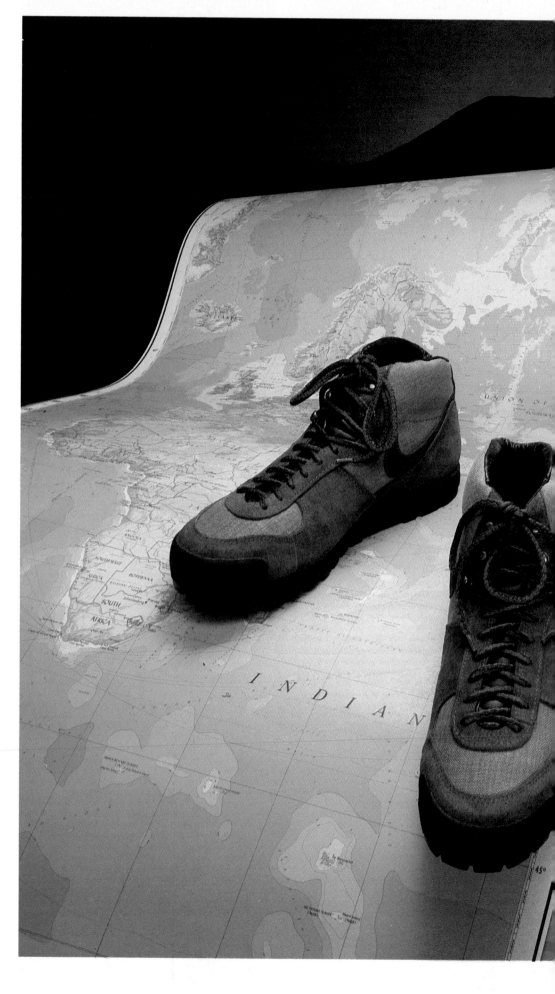

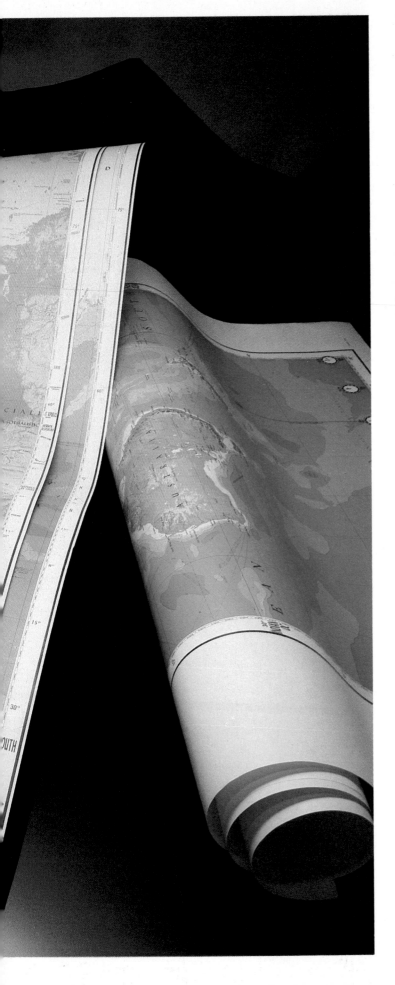

Fitness to Go

It's vacation time—time
for rejuvenation. Discover
the thrill of a fitness adventure!

"Because it's there," the ill-fated mountaineer G. L. Mallory said when asked why he wished to climb Mt. Everest. Mallory later vanished up there, in the mist above 26,000 feet, and only his ice-axe was ever found. But his comment has become the rallying cry of generations of bedazzled adventurers at a loss to explain why they do what they do.

Why *do* people decide—instead of spending their holiday in a deck chair—to dive the coral forests of the Cayman Islands, bike through China, trek beyond timberline in the Sierra Nevadas or confront the wilderness alone with nothing but their gumption and a minimum of tools?

It's the Mallory in them, certainly. But the rewards of taking a vacation that's a real physical effort rather than merely a rest aren't as hard to explain as the urge to climb a mountain. There's the excitement of anticipating a great trip—a bike tour of the California wine country, say—and using that as a powerful motivator for getting in shape. There's the satisfaction of testing your strength and stamina against a respectable fitness challenge, and coming up a winner. The sense that the places you see on your trip, you've *earned*. The pure, sensuous pleasure of putting your body through its paces. And that delicious "good tired" feeling at the end of a long, active day.

A "fitness vacation" may well turn out to be the most rewarding and memorable holiday you've ever taken. And with the great renaissance of interest in fitness, there's an extraordinary number of organized trips from which to choose, from inn-to-inn bicycle touring in Vermont to dive trips in the Caymans, at reasonable cost and with all the details taken care of. Or you can organize your own trip, at your own level of fitness, to your own Shangri-la. Think of it as a self-awarded blue ribbon—the delightful grand prize for a life of staying fit.

Bicycle Touring

Where to Begin

Bicycling magazine is a good place to begin your hunt for organized bike trips. If you're more interested in going it alone, the magazine also has published a series of small books called *Best Bicycle Tours* with recommended routes from California to Vermont.

"Try a vacation that's as good for your body as it is for your soul," is the slogan of one bike touring group. And it's true: On a bicycling vacation, you earn the soul-expanding exhilaration of all that grand scenery by burning off up to 2,000 calories a day. Not bad.

You can organize your own trip (and carry your own gear) or join one of the many organized tours in the United States, Canada or abroad (with all details taken care of in advance, and a support van or "sagwagon" taking up the rear with supplies and/or a lift for tired riders). *Bicycling* magazine's managing editor, Susan Weaver, took a busman's holiday when she joined a group of 23 other enthusiasts for a three-week tour of France and Germany. She found it was "really a great way to go because of the camaraderie of the group and the friendly response of Europeans we met."

Her trip, organized by two professors, was rather ambitious: The travelers covered 850 to 900 miles, averaging around 50 miles a day. "It was really a great motivation to get in shape," she says. Though she's a runner and commutes to work by bike, Susan trained for the trip by riding about 75 to 150 miles a week for several months. For many people, 50 miles a day may be too rigorous a schedule. Even Susan admits it was a bit much: "Sometimes it was really aggravating to ride through a beautiful little town and not have time to stop." So pick a trip that's going at *your* pace.

You might even try giving the old bike vacation an interesting new twist: off-road riding on the new lightweight but sturdy, 15-gear "fat tire" bikes made to leave roads behind. "It's a great new sport," says Sarah Lister, who with her husband runs bike trips of up to a week into the high country of northern New Mexico and southern Arizona. "You don't have to be a marathon man to be able to do it," she insists. "We get riders of all levels of ability." Following dirt forest-service roads or no roads at all, the cyclists explore meadows, canyons and forests, riding through grass and gravel and even crossing streams. "You spend as much time off the bike as on it, looking at wildflowers, exploring, walking up to see some new overlook," Sarah says. "It's great!"

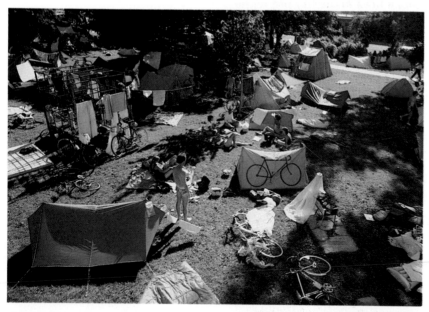

A bicycling vacation can be different things to different people. It can be an on-your-own excursion from inn to inn through the Vermont countryside, a serious tour with more competitive types or an organized camp-out among fun-loving enthusiasts.

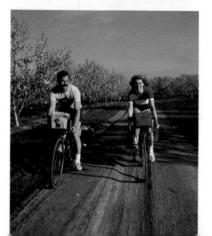

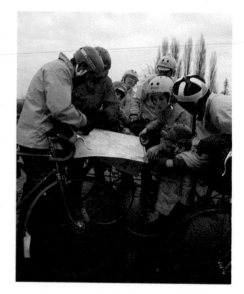

Running Camps

Want to combine the flavor of your childhood summer camp —the idyllic outdoor setting, the campfires and camaraderie—with no-nonsense training and special coaching aimed at making you a better runner? Then try a running camp.

For many runners, the chance to put in the miles on lovely forest trails rather than along smoggy highways is itself a major draw. Then there's the chance to meet and mingle with other runners, plus the "extras" like yoga, tennis, swimming, sailing and aerobic dance.

But what draws most runners is individualized coaching by experienced trainers (sometimes "big names" like Arthur Lydiard or Joan Ullyot, M.D.), the two or three supervised workouts a day and the lectures, on subjects ranging from nutrition and weight training to exercise physiology and new conditioning systems.

Coaching is what brought 49-year-old Gail Sangree to the Craftsbury Distance Running Camp in Craftsbury Common, Vermont. "I've run three marathons—slowly,"

she says. "I went to learn how to run faster." She was pleased with the running instruction she got, she says. "I was afraid it would be too much for me—all these young men with bulging muscles," says the teacher from Watertown, Connecticut, who didn't start running until she was 44. "But it really is good for people of all levels of ability."

Of course, you can take a vacation focused on running without attending a running camp at all. Los Angeles publicist Norman Conant does it by scheduling a ten-day pleasure trip to New York City every October—with the New York City Marathon sandwiched between sightseeing and shopping. He begins training in January—"that's when I know I'm serious," he says. He has a New York friend send him entry blanks and make hotel reservations around June, and he starts training in earnest by August. He spends at least a week in the city before the race and at least three days afterward to recover. But the marathon, he says, "is the high point of my trip."

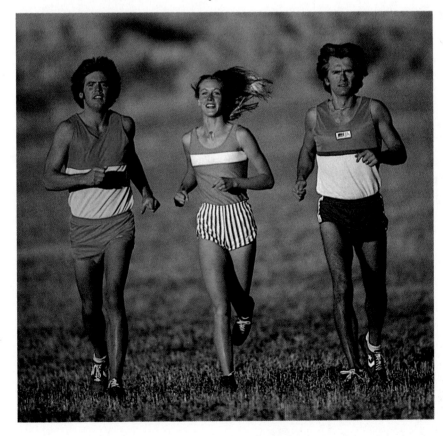

Take your vacation at a running camp this year and you'll experience the exhilarating lift of a heart-pumping workout in addition to breathtaking scenery. Many running camps are operated in captivating mountain country.

Mountain Hiking

Where to Begin

The popularity of backpacking in mountains here and abroad has spawned dozens of outfitters who organize, supply and lead trips. Information can be found in outdoor magazines like *Outside, Backpacker* or the Sierra Club's *Sierra.* You can get detailed topographical maps of most areas from the regional offices of the National Park Service or Forest Service.

"**I** can't think of a time I ever felt better, physically or mentally," says Takla Gardey, an editorial researcher from Pasadena, California, recalling the last days of her 21-day trek into the Himalaya Mountains of Nepal. "I just felt terrific. None of us wanted it to end."

It was the walking vacation of a lifetime, beginning outside Katmandu and following the main trading route (a well-worn footpath) between Tibet and Nepal up to 17,700 feet, then circling back again. In three weeks, the small group of trekkers walked 180 miles (8 to 12 miles a day), with Sherpa guides and porters who carried most of their gear and prepared meals.

"I was really concerned about being in shape for it, but the first few days went fairly slow so you got a chance to acclimatize," Takla says. "Actually, I underestimated my own stamina, as most people probably do. You don't really know what reserves you've got until you test them."

Hiking expeditions or "treks" to the Himalayas, the Alps or the Andes are becoming increasingly popular holidays for hikers who long to see the world—and *really* stretch their legs. But some of the most exhilarating mountain hiking in the world lies within the borders of the continental United States and Canada. Carol Mayernik, a dental assistant from Whitehall, Pennsylvania, read about "heli-hiking"—where intrepid hikers are flown into remote wilderness areas by helicopter—and decided to give it a try.

"It was a fabulous trip, worth every penny," she says, recalling her trip to an area of British Columbia's Purcell Mountains known as the Bugaboos. Her hiking group flew into the "base camp"—a luxurious lodge with first-class food and accommodations—and from there made daily trips into the mountains via a 14-passenger helicopter. Dropped off in trailless wilderness, they explored alpine meadows, glaciers and spectacular mountain forests. "When I got back, I felt so fit I thought I could do anything!" Carol laughs.

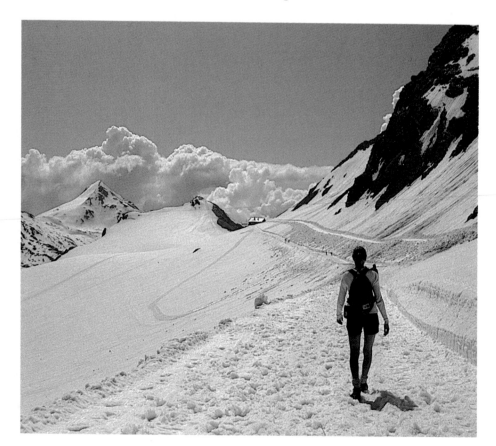

Sun *and* **snow-capped mountains. You can have it all, plus the peace and breathtaking view that can only be found by hiking above the clouds in the Swiss Alps.**

Trail Riding

"It was fabulous," says New York City economist Phil Rowland, recalling a four-day pack trip up to 8,000 feet in Wyoming's Absaroka Range, above Yellowstone National Park. "We rode up through conifer forest about 4 hours, then we broke out into an alpine meadow. We saw moose and eagles up there, and on nearby peaks there was snow—in August."

Riding a horse up through rugged, rocky terrain can be more strenuous than it looks, especially on the legs—and, of course, the derriere. "The first few days, you just get accustomed to being saddle sore," says Phil ruefully.

Mountain pack trips are a specialty at Grizzly Ranch, the "dude ranch" near Cody, Wyoming, where Phil and his family were spending their third vacation. Grizzly Ranch is a real working ranch where horses, mules and hay are raised and a small number of guests are taken in during the summer.

"Most of the activity here centers around riding," says Candy Felts, who runs the place with her husband, Rick, a former rodeo bareback rider. Besides pack trips, there are morning, afternoon and day-long rides (always led by a wrangler), and the opportunity to pitch in with ranch chores if you wish. There's also fishing, rafting, tennis and the ever-popular night rodeo in Cody.

Many dude ranches are like the Grizzly: actual working ranches where a few guests are taken in and made to feel like a part of the family. Others, sometimes called guest ranches, are primarily in the business of entertaining guests. They can often accommodate 15 to 50 visitors and may offer—along with riding, of course—amenities like heated swimming pools, square dances, barbecues, hay rides and programs for youngsters.

But the backwoods experience isn't limited to the wild West. Working farms from Wisconsin to Maine take in guests longing for a taste of the country life—from gathering eggs, picking vegetables or pitching hay to doing absolutely nothing at all.

Where to Begin

An excellent source of information about dude ranches and working farms is *Farm, Ranch & Country Vacations,* by Pat Dickerman. It will tell you all the specifics you need to know: directions, rates and accommodations, as well as a little bit about the *feeling* of the places.

For a taste of the old wild West, try a fitness vacation on a dude ranch. By day you might travel by horseback into the desert. At night, it's rest and relaxation by a ranch-style campfire.

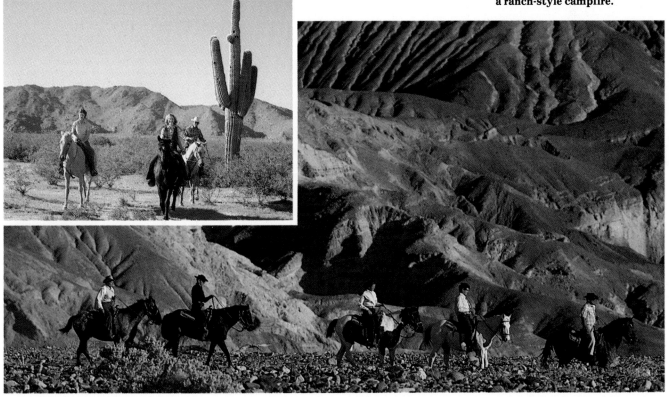

Scuba Diving

"If you're fit enough to play two sets of tennis and you've got your scuba certification, you're ready for a diving vacation in the Caribbean," says veteran dive instructor Steve Dee. "Advances in equipment over the past five or ten years have reduced the physical demands of sport diving considerably—you no longer have to be an exceptional swimmer, for instance, and you don't have to tread water for long periods of time. The hardest part about diving is carrying your equipment to the beach or the boat!"

You *do* need to know your physical limits, though, and you do need to keep your diving skills up to date. "Diving isn't like riding a bicycle," Steve says. "You tend to lose your skills if you don't use them. So if you haven't been in the water for nine months to a year, you need to get checked out again before heading out on a dive trip."

But the payoff for keeping your diving skills sharp and your body fit is tremendous. It may *look* like a Jacques Cousteau television special, but it's not: It's really *you* ghosting through the awesome world of a living coral reef, a weightless astronaut on an undersea planet as exotic and unworldly as the moon. It's an experience worth a great deal of trouble, training and expense.

Many Caribbean resorts cater specifically to divers, renting compressed air and all equipment, with dive boats going out up to three times a day. On a week-long dive trip, you could make 12 to 18 individual dives and still have time left over to sun, bike or swim. The best Caribbean dive spots are generally far from busy tourist areas like Nassau or Freeport, and, as a result, there isn't much night life—except for night dives on the reef, which can be the most thrilling dives of all. (Exceptions: Cozumel, Mexico, and the Cayman Islands both have good diving and are also popular nondivers' resorts.)

You don't have to leave the U.S. to find great warm-water diving, though. One favorite spot is the only living coral reef in North America, which runs for over 200 miles parallel to the Florida Keys, about 10 or 12 miles offshore.

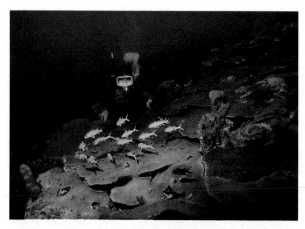

You can have your Caribbean island and exercise, too, by combining your sun and fun on a scuba-diving vacation.

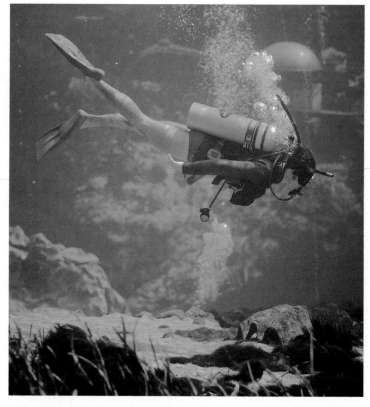

Survival Camps

What *would* you do if you got lost without food or shelter, alone, in the wilderness? It's a question many people ask themselves; only a daring (or unlucky) few have actually found out. Now you can get the experience, minus much of the terror, in wilderness survival schools across the United States and abroad.

Though Outward Bound is the best known, many other such schools now offer courses designed to teach people how to survive in every kind of environment and climate. The longer courses (they last from a few days to a month) often include the classic situation: you, alone, with a minimum of tools. Others teach all manner of survival skills, including "orienteering" (finding your way along an unfamiliar course), emergency first aid, learning the edible and medicinal plants, rock climbing, whitewater paddling, caving and even igloo building (in winter survival courses). Most programs teach low-impact camping and ecological awareness; they're also physically demanding enough to satisfy your urge to exercise.

"We started our morning with a brisk run and then we jumped in the ocean," says Barbara Reese, recalling the time she took from her studies at Pennsylvania State University to take part in an Outward Bound program on Hurricane Island, off the coast of Maine. Since it was October at the time, the ocean plunge was always a shock—and always brief. Although her course did not include an isolation period, Barbara did learn rock climbing, rappelling (descent by rope), sailing—and something about herself.

"The people who got the most out of it were those who didn't think they could do it—people like me, who were afraid to climb an 8-foot ladder and then found themselves hanging off a 100-foot rock," she says.

The course did not require an extraordinary level of fitness, she says—the group leader was a fit 55—but older people (especially those who have been inactive) might need to train to prepare themselves. The rewards for doing so are great: Many "outdoor" survival skills— courage, self-reliance, simplicity— work just as well indoors, and are of value whether or not you ever really *do* get lost in the wilderness.

Where to Begin

Specifics about wilderness survival schools like Outward Bound can usually be found in the classified section of outdoor publications like *Outside, Backpacker* or *Sierra.* Another good information source is the *Worldwide Adventure Travel Guide,* published yearly by the American Adventurers Association.

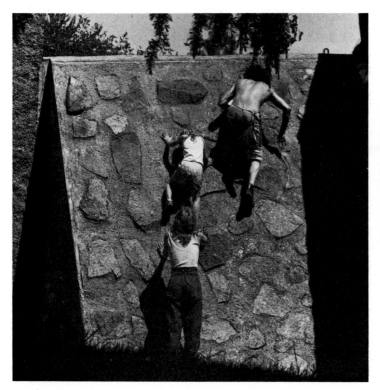

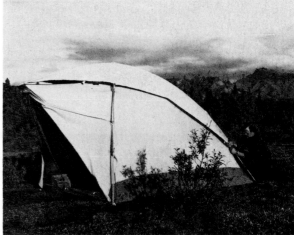

From a team effort in overcoming obstacles to living alone in the wilderness, survival training can be the ultimate in getting-away-from-it-all experiences.

Source Notes

Chapter 1
Page 9

"Age Doesn't Matter—If You Exercise" adapted from "Cardiorespiratory Health, Reaction Time and Aging," by David E. Sherwood and Dennis J. Selder in *Medicine and Science in Sports*, vol. 11, no. 2, 1979. Reprinted by permission of the publisher and authors.

Chapter 2
Page 18

"A Photo Finish" compiled from information from *Track and Field News* and the National Running Data Center.

Page 19

"The Warning Signs of Trouble" adapted from *The Cardiologists' Guide to Fitness and Health through Exercise*, by L. Zohman, M.D., A. A. Kattus, M.D. and D. G. Softness (New York: Simon & Schuster, 1979).

Chapter 4
Page 53

"Male Strong Points" compiled from information from the U. S. Weightlifting Federation and Judy Glenney.

Chapter 9
Page 145

"Sports Take Their Toll on the Knees" adapted from "Treatment of Injuries to Athletes: Special Problems of Runners and Joggers," by James D. Key (Dallas, Tex.: James D. Key, Sports Medicine Clinics of America, Key Clinic Associated, 1978). Reprinted by permission of the author.

Photography Credits

Cover: Margaret Skrovanek.
Staff Photographers—
Christopher Barone: pp. 5; 12-13; 51; 119; 128, top left, bottom left and top right; 130; 157. Angelo M. Caggiano: pp. 15; 142-143. Carl Doney: pp. 103; 132; 135. T. L. Gettings: pp. 8; 31, center right; 86; 95; 96; 97; 158, center right. John P. Hamel: pp. 7; 17. Ed Landrock: pp. 88; 90; 91; 92; 93. Mitchell T. Mandel: pp. 21; 29; 32; 36; 38; 40; 43; 45; 48-49; 57; 58; 59; 60; 61; 62; 63; 65; 69; 76; 77; 78; 79; 80; 81; 83; 84; 85; 100; 101; 112; 113; 116-117. Pat Seip: pp. 54; 99. Margaret Skrovanek: pp. 1; 25; 30, center right; 31, center left; 73; 149. Christie C. Tito: pp. 11; 47; 111; 128, center. Sally Shenk Ullman: p. 158, center left and bottom.

Other Photographers—
Mark Bricklin: p. 160. Tom Campbell: p. 161, center. Chuck Covko: p. 94, center. Bruce Faust: p. 94, bottom left. David Frazier: pp. 114; 115. P. Gridley: pp. 30-31, top. Dennis Hallinan: p. 162, bottom right. Russell Kelly: p. 159. Michael W. Koenig: p. 127. Richard Mackson: pp. 6; 52. Jeffrey W. Meyers: p. 163, bottom left. C. Roessler: p. 162, bottom left. Hubert Schriebl: p. 94, center left and center right. Irene Vandermolen: p. 163, bottom right. Joseph F. Viesti: p. 74. Jerry Wachter: pp. 26-27. Thomas Zimmerman: pp. 31, bottom right; 161, bottom.

*Additional Photos Courtesy of—*The Bettman Archive, N.Y.: pp. 34, bottom; 146. Focus on Sports: pp. 34, top right; 151. National Aeronautics and Space Administration: p. 64.

Illustration Credits

Susan Blubaugh: pp. 18; 20; 23; 55; 67; 70-71; 98-99, bottom; 107; 120-121; 122-123; 150; 153. Joe Lertola: pp. 28; 30; 32; 33; 34; 36; 37; 38; 40; 41; 42; 43; 44; 45; 46; 47; 48; 49; 86; 87; 88; 90; 91; 92, top left; 93; 94; 95, top right; 96, top left; 97, top right; 98, top right; 100; 124-125; 126-127; 139. Anita Lovitt: pp. 16; 35; 56; 82; 92, bottom right; 95, bottom left; 96, bottom right; 105; 129; 133; 140; 154; 155. Jerry O'Brien: p. 108; Donna Ruff: pp. 2; 3; 9; 39; 53; 75; 86; 97, bottom left; 106; 110; 136; 152.

Special Thanks to—
A & H Sporting Goods, Emmaus, Pa.; Converse, Inc., Wilmington, Md.; Elite Sportswear Ltd./ Gym-Kin, Reading, Pa.; Everything Goes, Inc., Whitehall, Pa.; Glori-Us Sportswear Ltd., Reading, Pa.; Nautilus Fitness Center, Allentown, Pa.; Nestor Sporting Goods, Whitehall, Pa.; Orthopaedic Associates of Allentown, Allentown, Pa.; Raven Industries, Inc., Sioux Falls, S.D.; Wilderness Travel Outfitters, Whitehall, Pa.

Index

Rodale Press, Inc., publishes PREVENTION®, the better health magazine.
For information on how to order your subscription,
write to PREVENTION®, Emmaus, PA 18049.